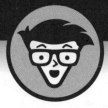

W9-BKQ-840

Vaccines

by Megan Coffee, MD, PhD,
and Sharon Perkins, RN

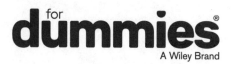

for
dummies®
A Wiley Brand

Vaccines For Dummies®

Published by: **John Wiley & Sons, Inc.,** 111 River Street, Hoboken, NJ 07030-5774, www.wiley.com

Copyright © 2021 by John Wiley & Sons, Inc., Hoboken, New Jersey

Published simultaneously in Canada

Contents at a Glance

Introduction 1

Part 1: Getting Started with Vaccine Basics 5
CHAPTER 1: Focusing on Vaccine Fundamentals 7
CHAPTER 2: The (Non) Life of a Virus 17
CHAPTER 3: The Crowned Virus: Coronavirus 31
CHAPTER 4: Bacterial Bad Guys 57

Part 2: Verifying Valuable Vaccines 67
CHAPTER 5: Distinguishing and Testing Different Vaccines 69
CHAPTER 6: Tracking the Current List of Effective Vaccines 85
CHAPTER 7: What to Expect When You're Vaccinating 105

Part 3: Scheduling Safety 123
CHAPTER 8: Vaccines for Children 125
CHAPTER 9: Vaccines for Adults 147
CHAPTER 10: Spelling Out Who May Face Risks 161
CHAPTER 11: Anti-Vaxxers and Debunking Myths About Vaccines 175

Part 4: The Part of Tens 191
CHAPTER 12: Five People Who Created Ten (Or More) Modern Vaccines 193
CHAPTER 13: Ten Diseases Without Vaccines, from A to Z 199
CHAPTER 14: The Ten Most Lethal Major Pandemics 211
CHAPTER 15: Ten Ways to Boost Your Immune System 219

Index 225

Table of Contents

INTRODUCTION 1
- About This Book. 1
- Foolish Assumptions. 2
- Icons Used in This Book 2
- Beyond the Book 2
- Where to Go from Here 3

PART 1: GETTING STARTED WITH VACCINE BASICS 5

CHAPTER 1: Focusing on Vaccine Fundamentals 7
- Realizing the Crucial Role of Vaccines 8
- Explaining How a Vaccine Works. 9
  - Distinguishing between antigens and antibodies. 10
  - Breaking down other vaccine ingredients 10
- Comparing Viruses, Bacteria, and Toxins 11
- Studying COVID-19 Vaccine Development. 14
- Understanding the Importance of Vaccine Schedules. 15
- Preparing for Potential Vaccine Side Effects 16
- Optimizing Your Immune Response. 16

CHAPTER 2: The (Non) Life of a Virus 17
- Looking Inside Your Average Virus 18
- Investigating Influenza Viruses 18
  - Type A 19
  - Type B 21
  - Type C 21
  - Type D 22
- Examining Enteroviruses (Including Rhinoviruses). 22
- Knowing About Norovirus 23
- Understanding HIV 24
- Trying to Say Goodbye to Measles 25
- Checking Out the Cause of Chicken Pox: Varicella 26
- Fighting Ebola. 27
- Surveying Variola (Smallpox) 29

CHAPTER 3: The Crowned Virus: Coronavirus 31
- Identifying the Coronavirus in Humans 32
- Combatting the Common Cold Coronavirus 33
  - What is a cold, exactly? 34
  - What causes a cold? 34
  - When is a cold not a cold? 35

Surveying SARS and MERS 40
    Severe acute respiratory syndrome (SARS) .40
    Middle East respiratory syndrome (MERS) 41
COVID-19: The Novel (and Specially Confounding) Coronavirus 42
    Reviewing the start of the pandemic 42
    Charting the course of the infection 44
    Detecting a COVID-19 infection 46
    Digging into the development of COVID-19 vaccines 50
    Dealing with vaccine side effects 52
    Aiming for herd immunity 53
    Keeping safe from COVID-19 if you're not yet protected
    by vaccination 55
    Coping with COVID-19 and flu season 56

CHAPTER 4: **Bacterial Bad Guys** 57
Understanding What Makes Bacteria Different from Viruses 57
Digging into Vaccines That Defuse Bacteria 58
    The make-up of vaccines that protect against bacterial toxins 59
    The bacterial illnesses that vaccines prevent 59
Comparing Antibiotics and Vaccines 64
Seeing How Vaccines Help Prevent Antibiotic Resistance 65

PART 2: VERIFYING VALUABLE VACCINES 67

CHAPTER 5: **Distinguishing and Testing Different Vaccines** 69
Getting to Know the Different Types of Vaccines 70
    Whole-pathogen vaccines 70
    Subunit vaccines 72
Testing Vaccines for Safety and Effectiveness 75
    Determining the need and costs: The preclinical stage 75
    Phase I 76
    Phase II 76
    Phase III 76
    Post–Phase III 77
Studying the Efficacy of Vaccines 78
    Measuring efficacy versus effectiveness 78
    Rounding up herd immunity 79
Tracing the History of Various Vaccines 80
    Smallpox 80
    Typhoid fever 81
    Yellow fever 81
    Influenza 82
    Polio 82
    Anthrax 82
    Measles, mumps, and rubella (MMR) 82
    Varicella (chicken pox) 83

CHAPTER 6: **Tracking the Current List of Effective Vaccines** 85

Chicken Pox (Varicella) 85

Diphtheria, Tetanus, and Pertussis................................86

    Diphtheria..86

    Tetanus 87

    Pertussis 88

Haemophilus Influenzae Type B (Hib) 88

Hepatitis A 89

Hepatitis B 90

Human Papillomavirus (HPV).....................................92

Influenza (Flu)..93

Measles, Mumps, and Rubella (MMR) 95

Measles, Mumps, Rubella, and Varicella (MMRV)................97

Meningococcal Vaccines...97

Pneumococcal Vaccines 98

    For adults 99

    For children 100

Rotavirus...101

Shingles (Herpes Zoster)..102

CHAPTER 7: **What to Expect When You're Vaccinating** 105

Understanding Side Effects: What May Cause Them and
What Happens 106

    Looking at common vaccine ingredients 106

    Distinguishing vaccine delivery methods.....................110

    Watching for localized skin reactions........................111

    Expecting a systemic immune response 114

Recognizing and Treating Serious Reactions......................116

    Avoiding allergic reactions 117

    Anaphylactic reactions 117

    Febrile seizures after childhood vaccinations.................118

    Guillain-Barré syndrome 119

    Thrombocytopenia 120

Looking at Multiple Vaccines and the Immune System...........120

PART 3: SCHEDULING SAFETY..................................123

CHAPTER 8: **Vaccines for Children** 125

Understanding Mom-to-Baby Immunity 125

    Breastfeeding benefits 126

    Antibodies passed on during pregnancy.....................126

Getting a Reminder of the Effectiveness and Importance of
Vaccinations 127

Focusing on Vaccinations in the First Year of Life................127

    Hepatitis B 128

    Rotavirus..129

DTaP (Diphtheria, tetanus, pertussis)...........................131
Hib..132
IPV (inactivated polio vaccine)................................132
Influenza..133
PCV13..134
Knowing New Vaccinations for Toddlers..........................134
MMR (measles, mumps, rubella)..................................136
Varicella or MMRV..139
Hepatitis A..140
Surveying a Few Vaccines for Ages 4 to 6.......................140
Adding Some School-Age Vaccinations............................141
Human papillomavirus (HPV).....................................141
Meningococcal conjugate (MenACWY)..............................142
Tetanus, diphtheria, and pertussis (Tdap)......................142
Needing a Booster: Vaccines for Teens..........................143
Catching Up on Childhood Vaccines..............................144
Spreading vaccines out...144
Starting vaccines late...144
Adopting a child from another country..........................145
Checking Out Vaccine Schedules Around the World................146

CHAPTER 9: **Vaccines for Adults**............................147
Vaccines When You're 19–26 Years Old...........................147
Your yearly flu shot...148
The COVID-19 vaccine...149
A Tdap or Td booster...150
Vaccines When You're 27–49 Years Old...........................151
Vaccines When You're 50–64 Years Old...........................151
Vaccines When You're 65-Plus Years Old.........................153
Influenza..153
Tdap...155
Pneumococcal vaccines..156
Vaccines Before and During Pregnancy...........................156
Vaccines for Travelers...157
Making sure you're up to date on routine vaccines..............158
Getting other vaccines depending on your destination...........158
Catching Up: If Your Parents/Guardians Didn't Vaccinate You....160

CHAPTER 10: **Spelling Out Who May Face Risks**...............161
Knowing When to Avoid or Limit Vaccines........................161
Considering vaccines and cancer................................162
Vaccines and immune disorders..................................163
Vaccines after organ transplantation...........................164

Understanding Vaccines and Allergies...........................165
    Allergies to vaccine ingredients and components 165
    Different types of reactions..................................168
    Recognizing reactions that actually aren't allergies 169
    Taking precautions before vaccination 169
Assessing Reactions to the COVID-19 Vaccine 170
    Rare cases of anaphylaxis 170
    Other types of reactions.....................................170
    Inspecting ingredients found in current COVID-19 vaccines.....171
    Getting the COVID-19 vaccine after you've had COVID-19 173

CHAPTER 11: Anti-Vaxxers and Debunking Myths About Vaccines...175
Studying the Rise of Vaccine Hesitancy 176
    Understanding why some people don't vaccinate 176
    Looking at the early anti-vaxxers 178
Debunking Common Vaccine Myths............................179
    Myth: Diseases were disappearing before vaccines were invented 180
    Myth: Vaccines cause serious side effects, illnesses, and death.......................................180
    Myth: Kids don't need to be vaccinated so young 181
    Myth: Kids don't need to be vaccinated when illnesses don't exist in their country...................................184
    Myth: Giving multiple vaccines at the same time overloads the immune system..184
    Myth: Vaccines can cause the disease they are supposed to prevent...185
    Myth: Not getting vaccinated affects only me.................186
    Myth: Natural immunity is always best 186
    Myth: The MMR vaccine causes autism 187
    Myth: Vaccines contain harmful chemicals 188
Reviewing Vaccine Recalls 189

PART 4: THE PART OF TENS...................................191

CHAPTER 12: Five People Who Created Ten (Or More) Modern Vaccines 193
Edward Jenner: Snuffing Out Smallpox 193
Louis Pasteur: Ridding the World of Rabies......................194
Jonas Salk and Albert Sabin: Putting Polio Behind Us 195
Maurice Hilleman: The Master of Modern Vaccines..............196

CHAPTER 13: **Ten Diseases Without Vaccines, from A to Z** 199

Avian Influenzas (Bird Flu) 200
Cytomegalovirus (CMV). 200
Epstein-Barr Virus (EBV) 201
Hepatitis C 202
Herpes Simplex Virus (HSV) 1 and 2 203
HIV/AIDS 204
Lyme Disease. 205
Respiratory Syncytial Virus (RSV). 207
West Nile Virus. 208
Zika Virus 209

CHAPTER 14: **The Ten Most Lethal Major Pandemics** 211

Antonine Plague (165–180) 212
Plague of Justinian (541–750). 212
Bubonic Plague (Black Death) (1346–1353) 213
Cholera (1846–1860). 214
Third Plague Pandemic (1855–1960) 215
Influenza (Russian Flu) (1889–1890). 215
Influenza (Spanish Flu) (1918–1919). 216
Influenza (Asian Flu) (1957–1958) 217
Human Immunodeficiency Virus (HIV) (1981–Present) 217
COVID-19 (2020–Present). 218

CHAPTER 15: **Ten Ways to Boost Your Immune System** 219

Getting Your Vaccinations 219
Decreasing Stress 220
Eating Well 220
Maintaining a Healthy Weight 221
Getting Enough Sleep 221
Exercising for Immunity 222
Saying No to Smoking. 222
Drinking Only in Moderation 223
Staying Connected. 223
Considering Supplements 224

INDEX 225

Introduction

Vaccines are a hot topic today, but that's really not anything new. They have been lauded, criticized, and discussed for hundreds of years, although the creation of new vaccines has certainly accelerated over the past 70 or so years. Yet dozens of misconceptions about vaccines still exist. For every person who embraces being fully vaccinated, there's someone who questions certain vaccines or, worse, rejects them altogether, despite their proven benefits.

This book is for both groups — the people who vaccinate themselves and their families but who want to know more about them, and the people who have questions about vaccines. Our goal is to have everyone vaccinated and, even more important, happy knowing they're doing the best thing for their health.

About This Book

Obviously, vaccines are the main topic of this book. But we intend to do more than just give you a vaccine schedule. We explain the history of vaccines (and it goes back much further than you might think), talk about the types of germs and diseases that led to vaccine development, and explain why the vaccine schedules are set up the way they are. We also discuss the myths about vaccines, especially with regard to children, and explain why the vaccine schedules have changed over the years.

A quick note: Sidebars (shaded boxes of text) dig into the details of a given topic, but they aren't crucial to understanding it. Feel free to read them or skip them. You can pass over the text accompanied by the Technical Stuff icon, too. The text marked with this icon gives some interesting but nonessential information about vaccines.

One last thing: Within this book, you may note that some web addresses break across two lines of text. If you're reading this book in print and want to visit one of these web pages, simply key in the web address exactly as it's noted in the text, pretending as though the line break doesn't exist. If you're reading this as an e-book, you've got it easy — just click the web address to be taken directly to the web page.

Foolish Assumptions

Here are some assumptions about you, dear reader, and why you're picking up this book:

>> You want to learn more about vaccines in general.

>> You're willing to keep an open mind about vaccines and vaccinations.

>> You're looking for more information about how vaccines are created.

>> You have questions about vaccine scheduling.

Icons Used in This Book

Like all *For Dummies* books, this book features icons to help you navigate the information. Here's what they mean.

If you take away anything from this book, it should be the information marked with this icon.

REMEMBER

This icon flags information that delves a little deeper than usual into a particular topic related to vaccines.

TECHNICAL STUFF

This icon highlights especially helpful advice about vaccines and vaccinations.

TIP

This icon points out situations and actions to avoid when you're planning to be vaccinated.

WARNING

Beyond the Book

In addition to the material in the print or e-book you're reading right now, this product comes with some access-anywhere goodies on the web. Check out the free Cheat Sheet for questions to ask your pediatrician about vaccines, facts about adult vaccinations, and the scoop on different types of vaccines. To get this Cheat Sheet, simply go to www.dummies.com and search for "Vaccines For Dummies Cheat Sheet" in the Search box.

Where to Go from Here

You don't have to read this book from cover to cover, but if you're an especially thorough person, feel free to do so! If you just want to find specific information and then get back to work, take a look at the table of contents or the index, and then dive into the chapter or section that interests you.

For example, if you're just looking for more information on childhood vaccination schedules, go to Chapter 8. Adult schedules are in Chapter 9. If side effects concern you, read Chapter 7. And if your main interest right now is coronaviruses, you'll find a ton of info in Chapter 3.

Vaccines have changed the world for the better. We hope this book gives you confidence that vaccinating yourself and your family is the best way to keep you all healthy.

1
Getting Started with Vaccine Basics

IN THIS PART . . .

Focus on the fundamentals of vaccines.

Investigate viruses — what they are and how they work.

Understand coronaviruses from colds to COVID-19.

Get a handle on defeating dangerous bacteria.

IN THIS CHAPTER

» Looking at the importance of vaccines

» Getting a handle on how vaccines work

» Surveying the COVID-19 vaccine

» Checking out schedules and side effects

» Boosting your immune system's response

Chapter **1**

Focusing on Vaccine Fundamentals

Infections that once haunted childhood are now seen only in textbooks. These were the true bogeymen of childhood, the real monsters under the bed. They were common and potentially life-threatening. We now have vaccines for these infections that were so tricky to treat and easy to spread. Most children around the world are vaccinated against these bogeymen, including, among others, measles, polio, diphtheria, tetanus, and smallpox. Vaccines have helped send these diseases packing, even though we still don't always have good treatments for the diseases themselves.

There's a lot of information — and misinformation — out there about vaccines. When large groups lose trust in the benefits of vaccination, many people, not just those who don't want to be vaccinated, can suffer. Diseases like COVID-19 can continue to spread. Those who have weakened immune systems that don't respond well to vaccines can be infected by others. It's important that we keep our eyes on the common enemy — infectious diseases.

Realizing the Crucial Role of Vaccines

Vaccinations provide a valuable tool. You can give your immune system a heads-up about infections before you ever see them. You can stop diseases before you ever get sick by giving your immune system a cheat sheet on what to look for. Unlike medications that reduce the symptoms once the illness has begun, vaccines can stop infections before they ever happen. Childhood — and adulthood — have become a lot safer in the process.

Vaccines give your immune system a superpower. Through vaccines, your immune system learns how to stop bad guys it's never seen before. These bad guys cause infectious diseases. They're the *pathogens,* also called germs, which are so tiny that we can see them only with a microscope. These pathogens include bacteria, viruses, fungi, and parasites. Chapter 2 describes different viruses and the vaccines that combat them, while bacteria and their vaccines are discussed in Chapter 4.

REMEMBER

Vaccines provide you with personal protection against these pathogens and the diseases they cause, but what works even better is if everyone is vaccinated. The superpower of a vaccine increases as more people jump on the bandwagon. With infectious diseases, we're all in this together. If everyone is vaccinated, a pathogen spreading person to person is stymied.

Vaccines may not provide 100 percent protection. Some people may not be able to take or benefit from a vaccine; they may be too young or have a weakened immune system. But if enough of us are vaccinated, odds are the pathogen just can't spread. It can't jump from person to person. It may infect one person and maybe another, but if most people are vaccinated, it won't keep finding new people to spread to and will fade away.

This is what *herd immunity* is all about — when enough people are vaccinated, we can push back the spread of some terrible and deadly diseases. Chapter 11 details the benefits of herd immunity and debunks the myths often perpetuated about vaccines. Diseases can bounce back if fewer people are vaccinated.

We can save many lives if we had more vaccines. Scientific challenges and the lack of funding and motivation have kept some vaccines from being developed. (See Chapter 13 for more information.) New diseases yet to emerge will need vaccines, as we have seen as COVID-19 has spread around the world. (See Chapter 3 for info on COVID-19 and the vaccine.)

It may not seem so exciting now, but we have had reliable and effective vaccines only since the end of the 1700s. At that time, it was found that one mild virus, cowpox, can train our immune system to protect us from a terrible virus, smallpox. (If vaccine history interests you, check out Chapter 12, which discusses the people instrumental in creating a number of vaccines. Chapter 14 describes major pandemics throughout history.)

Many vaccines work on the same principle as this first vaccine did: Show the immune system something harmless but similar to what causes the disease, and the immune system will learn to protect us against the dangerous one too. However, scientists continue working on vaccines to develop new, possibly more effective approaches to train our immune system. Different pathogens require different sorts of vaccines, and for some diseases, vaccines still elude us.

We do have vaccines for a wide range of infections, though. Vaccines can prevent some types of liver disease (hepatitis A and B) and some types of cancer (human papillomavirus). We also have vaccines for adults, such as for pneumonias and shingles, diseases we're more prone to as we get older. But we still don't have vaccines for the infections that year after year take the most lives. We don't have an HIV vaccine, and we need better vaccines for tuberculosis and malaria. We also don't have a vaccine for the common cold, which would be hard to make. Chapter 6 provides information on all current vaccines, while Chapter 13 looks at diseases that still aren't preventable.

REMEMBER

As is often said about vaccines, it's not vaccines that save lives; it's vaccinations. For communities to be protected, vaccines need to be given. The tough part is often ensuring that vaccines are accessible for all and vaccination rates are high enough to protect the entire community.

Explaining How a Vaccine Works

Vaccines hold up a "Wanted" photo of the bad guy — the pathogen or germ. Each vaccine is a little different, but they all show our immune system something super recognizable about the pathogen. That way, if we are ever exposed to this pathogen, our immune systems will respond to it.

The "Wanted" photo can be some bit from the outside of the pathogen, like a specific protein or sugar. These bits act as a way to identify the pathogen, similar to the way a tattoo or birthmark helps you identify a person. The vaccine version may attach this "Wanted" photo to a warning, like a blinking red light, such as a protein that will create a stronger immune response.

Other vaccines may be the equivalent of a head-to-foot photo; some vaccines use the whole pathogen (in a killed vaccine, explained more in Chapter 5) or in a live, but safe, similar version. Chapter 7 discusses the ingredients that typically make up vaccines.

Vaccines let you bypass the delay it would take to develop natural immunity if you were first exposed to the pathogen without this head start. Normally, it can take a couple of weeks for your immune system to figure out how to fight a new disease; with a vaccine, your body is ready and able to fight from the first time you see the actual pathogen.

Find out more about the basics of how a vaccine works in the following sections.

Distinguishing between antigens and antibodies

Antigens are what is memorable in the "Wanted" photo. An antigen is something very specific — like that birthmark or tattoo — that can't be missed. Your immune system uses that very specific marking to create an immune response and memory. This marking is usually a protein or sometimes a sugar on the outside of the pathogen.

Antibodies are what your body makes in response to antigens. After your body has been shown the antigen or "Wanted" photo, you keep a supply of memory immune cells that can make a whole lot more antibodies if the pathogen ever arrives. Specific antibodies go after just one specific antigen. Once that antigen is found again, your body floods it with copies of this antibody from those memory immune cells. The antibodies then attach themselves to their antigens, which are on the outside of the pathogen. The antibodies then stop this specific pathogen, like a virus particle or bacterium cell, from causing any more problems.

It typically takes a few weeks after exposure for the body to produce this response. Vaccination gives you a head start so you already have the ability to make all these antibodies if you need to. With a natural infection, you can get quite sick before you were able to scramble and create an effective immune response.

Breaking down other vaccine ingredients

Vaccines contain more than just the "Wanted" photos, called antigens, that help your immune system identify pathogens (see the preceding section). Other ingredients are needed to make sure the vaccine works as it should:

>> Some of these "Wanted" photos don't create much of an immune response. The immune system needs to be alerted to the fact that this "Wanted" photo is important to remember. Vaccines may include an alert, which acts like a red blinking light, saying "pay attention here." This ingredient may even be directly attached to the "Wanted" photo. Such alerts when added to the vaccine mix

are called *adjuvants*. A common adjuvant includes aluminum, also found in drinking water, antacids, and antiperspirants. We discuss the ingredients that go into vaccines more in Chapter 7.

» Vaccines also may contain stabilizers, much like some of our food does. These include sugars and gelatin (also found in Jell-O) that keep the vaccine ingredients well mixed, so they don't separate or deteriorate.

» Vaccines can sometimes include preservatives to keep mold or bacteria from growing in the vaccine, much like we would have in a bottle of jam at home. Just as many foods are advertised as preservative-free, many vaccines are too. Preservatives are particularly used in multi-use vaccine bottles, especially for the flu, as these are kept open longer to vaccinate multiple people. In some cases, this can include thimerosal, which contains mercury, but it's a type of mercury that doesn't have the same worrisome risk as the mercury found in fish. Children's vaccines do not include mercury, except in rare cases with multi-use flu vaccine vials and some specific brands of tetanus shots for adolescents.

» Vaccines may also include trace amounts of chemicals used in their production. These substances are removed, but sometimes a very small amount remains. In order to include a whole virus or bacteria but make sure it's dead and won't make copies of itself, formaldehyde is used. The amount used in a vaccine is much, much less than we naturally have in our bodies.

» Sometimes antibiotics, usually not the sorts we are allergic to, are used to keep bacteria from growing during production. These antibiotics are removed at the end, so at most only a tiny amount remains. Eggs are used to grow some viruses used to make vaccines, and so egg proteins, in very tiny amounts, may be present in some specific vaccines.

Comparing Viruses, Bacteria, and Toxins

REMEMBER

Scientists have studied and created different vaccines for a whole range of different pathogens. Pathogens are the germs, so small that you need a microscope to see them, that cause infectious diseases. The two main types of pathogens we vaccinate against are viruses and bacteria:

» **Viruses** are super tiny particles, made of genetic material surrounded by a protein shell. They can make copies of themselves only inside of other cells.

» **Bacteria** are more complicated; they are single-celled, living organisms that can usually make copies of themselves on their own.

Viruses, the smallest of the common pathogens, are protein shells with a bit of genetic instructions tucked away inside. Viruses use these instructions inside another cell, such as our own, to make copies of themselves; in the process our cells may be damaged by the virus or our immune system's response. Because viruses can't make copies of themselves on their own and need to be inside a cell, they aren't considered fully alive. We go more in-depth about viruses in Chapter 2.

Pathogens also include bacteria, as we talk about in Chapter 4. These are made up of a single cell that can reproduce on its own. Some bacteria invade your cells; others remain outside; some may do either. You have lots of bacteria inside your body at any time. In fact, we have more bacterial cells than human cells in our bodies. Our skin and gut and immune systems keep these bacteria where they should be, but sometimes these bacteria or new invading bacteria can make you sick. Antibiotics can work against these worrisome bacteria, but antibiotics don't work as quickly as vaccines. Vaccines prevent you from ever getting sick, while antibiotics only reduce the symptoms once you do get sick.

Other types of pathogens include the following:

>> **Parasites:** These can be single-celled like malaria, which is a lot larger and more complicated than bacteria are. Parasites can also include worms that infect you or even tiny insects like bed bugs or scabies. We haven't been successful at making vaccines for many of these but are now having some success with making vaccines for malaria.

>> **Fungi:** These are effectively the mini cousins of mushrooms. They include molds and yeasts. Infections may be from the environment, say from a dust storm in Arizona that can spread Valley Fever, a fungal infection, from the sand and dust. There haven't been any approved fungal vaccines.

>> **Prions:** Like viruses, prions also aren't really alive, and they're even smaller. They're just crumped proteins that can cause other proteins of the same type to crumple up in the same way. This type of infection causes Mad Cow Disease and a few other diseases, but they're incredibly rare. We don't yet have any vaccines for prion diseases in humans (but there is some promising work for animal diseases).

Vaccines for viruses and bacteria can include many different types (see Chapter 5 for details):

>> The oldest type is a similar but alive (or replicating) bacteria or virus that shows our immune system what the danger is without causing us any harm.

>> Another tried-and-true method is to take killed, whole bacteria or viruses. These won't be able to infect us but will show our immune system what to watch for.

>> Other vaccines use small proteins or sugars, found on the outside of bacteria or viruses, that can be used to recognize pathogens.

IS THIS INGREDIENT SAFE?

Vaccines go through rigorous multi-stage testing to ensure they prevent disease and are safe without worrisome side effects. Once vaccines are approved, they continue to be watched for any signs of any problems. Chapter 5 looks more closely at the vaccine testing and manufacturing processes.

The ingredients in vaccines are carefully monitored to ensure they don't have worrisome side effects. The ingredients are clearly listed in the insert that comes with the vaccine. If you ever have any questions about any ingredients and whether you might be allergic to one, you can discuss this with your doctor or healthcare provider.

After vaccines are approved by government agencies, including the Food and Drug Administration (FDA) in the United States, they are still monitored for any signs of problems. Anyone who is vaccinated in the United States can report any side effects to a national database that watches for and tracks patterns and serious events.

The manufacturing of vaccines is also watched closely. There are ongoing inspections and monitoring of vaccine production facilities by the FDA in the United States and by other independent government organizations in other countries. Around the world, the World Health Organization (WHO) also assesses factories before they begin production for quality, safety, and efficacy. Only factories that are continually inspected and approved for production can make the vaccines.

Once vaccines are produced, they undergo testing again. Vaccines are made in batches called *lots.* Samples from every single lot must be tested to ensure they have the pure, potent, and safe ingredients they are intended to have. No vaccine lot can be distributed until it is released by the FDA. Other countries have similar regulations. If a problem was found in a vaccine from one lot, the entire lot can be recalled.

Once vaccines are released, they have to be packaged and stored in certain conditions to keep the vaccine from deteriorating. Many vaccines require what is called *cold chain,* meaning they have to be kept within a very specific range of cold temperatures all the way from factory to delivery for vaccination. That way, you can feel assured that the vaccine you receive is still potent when you receive it.

>> Some vaccines are made against the toxins that bacteria release to make us sick. The vaccine includes something similar and benign, called *toxoids,* which don't make us sick, in order to teach our bodies to recognize toxins.

>> Two new types of vaccines have been used so far for viruses — viral vector vaccines and vaccines made from genetic material, like mRNA. These vaccines carry the genetic instructions into our cells in order to build a protein that our immune systems can use to recognize a pathogen.

Studying COVID-19 Vaccine Development

Infectious diseases have not been completely tamed. COVID-19 reminds us there are many viruses and bacteria out there that we've never dealt with before. It goes without saying that COVID-19 changed the world abruptly for us all. In the first full year of the pandemic (2020), it led to at least 350,000 deaths in the United States and at least 1.8 million deaths reported worldwide. Vaccines have been an important part of the solution.

No vaccines have been watched as closely as the COVID-19 vaccines as they passed through phase I, then II, then III, and onto use in the general population. The world watched as controlled trials studied the use of the vaccines versus a placebo. These trials — as well as post-rollout monitoring — looked closely for any side effects.

As we discuss in more detail in Chapter 3, many different types of vaccine methods are used today. A lot of advances in vaccine science led to the COVID-19 vaccines. The first vaccines came from science that was only a couple of decades old. The COVID-19 vaccines currently in use are messenger RNA (mRNA) or viral vector vaccines.

REMEMBER

Vaccines were also shown to provide better protection than natural infection, especially when facing new variants of COVID-19. As COVID-19 has spread around the globe, it has collected many new mutations creating new variants, so your immune system may not recognize new variants after getting sick with a prior one. It may become necessary to have booster COVID-19 vaccinations to remain immune, just like you need to remain protected against the flu.

WHY LAST YEAR'S FLU VACCINE WON'T WORK THIS YEAR

Most vaccines work well year after year. Some, particularly for influenza, need an update. That's because some pathogens change their looks. It's the pathogen equivalent of a wig or a fake moustache that fools our immune systems. What the pathogen looked like last year may not be what it looks like this year, at least to our immune systems.

Pathogens may change their looks by collecting mutations that each make small changes generation after generation. Over time, in a pathogen's family tree, the great-grandparents may look just a bit different than future generations. There may be different proteins (or sugars) on their surfaces, making them unrecognizable.

The flu does even more to dodge your immune system's attention. Mutations build up as the flu copies itself again and again. But it does something more. It also mixes and matches the proteins on the outside. It takes a fake moustache and a hat one year, a wig and a mask another year. This means a vaccine that works this year may not work next year. Some types may persist for a few years. Others need to be updated. As we discuss in Chapter 6, a lot of thought goes into the flu vaccine each year, trying to guess six months ahead which fake moustaches and wigs will be en vogue for the flu this year. The vaccine is updated every year in both the Northern and Southern hemispheres in time to vaccinate everyone who wants it in preparation for the wintertime flu season.

Understanding the Importance of Vaccine Schedules

Unfortunately, vaccines don't always fall into the "one and done" category. In many cases, a series of vaccines, given on a specific schedule, are necessary to provide you or your children with protection against diseases. While no one wants to get an injection more than once, skipping doses or spreading them out can decrease the effectiveness of the vaccine and increase your chance of becoming ill.

REMEMBER

Vaccine schedules are particularly important for infants and children because the diseases that the vaccines prevent are especially deadly for them. While the number of vaccines given to babies today has increased, worrying some parents, science has shown that the total number of vaccines given today isn't harmful. Spreading out vaccines on a delayed schedule can be harmful rather than helpful to infants, increasing their risk of becoming sick. To help you make the best decisions about vaccinations, Chapter 11 discusses the myths that surround vaccination and vaccine schedules, especially for young children.

Trying to keep track of vaccination schedules can be complicated. We make it easier by describing which vaccines are required for infants and children at which ages in Chapter 8. We include the same information for adults in Chapter 9. Chapter 10 explains when you or your child should *not* get vaccinated, due to certain health conditions. Thankfully, these conditions are rare.

Preparing for Potential Vaccine Side Effects

Any substance you put inside the human body has the potential to cause side effects. In most cases, side effects don't affect everyone, and most side effects aren't serious or long lasting. But it's always nice to be prepared for typical side effects, and it's important to be aware of more serious side effects that necessitate a visit to your healthcare provider. We spell out side effects and what to watch for in Chapter 7.

WARNING

Rarely, around one in a million or so cases, a vaccine can cause an anaphylactic reaction. This type of reaction can affect many body systems and be life-threatening. Anaphylactic reactions can occur if you have an allergy to one of the ingredients found in the vaccine. If you have known allergies to a vaccine or a possible vaccine component, always check the ingredients on a vaccine's label before being vaccinated. Anaphylactic reactions can include difficulty breathing, facial swelling, a drop in blood pressure, or loss of consciousness. Most, but not all, anaphylactic reactions occur within a few minutes after receiving a vaccine.

WARNING

Anaphylactic reactions are a medical emergency and require immediate medical attention. If you've had this type of reaction in the past, your healthcare provider may recommend carrying an epinephrine (epi) pen.

Optimizing Your Immune Response

REMEMBER

While you can't prevent all illnesses, you can do your part to keep your immune system as healthy and effective as possible. Getting vaccinated is the number one thing you can do to boost your immune system. Certain lifestyle changes can also help keep your immune system humming.

No, there are no magic bullets, pills, or other easy ways to do this. But Chapter 15 includes information that you may not have realized on ways to keep your immune system healthy, from the effects of smoking and alcohol on your immune system to the benefits of getting enough sleep. We also include info on supplements often taken for good health.

Chapter **2**

The (Non) Life of a Virus

You've probably said, "I caught a virus" dozens of times in your life. And no wonder — so far humans have identified close to 7,000 virus species. We know there are hundreds of thousands more and think there are millions, if not trillions, more. Some viruses infect people; others infect other animals; and still others infect plants, fungi, or even bacteria. (There are even *virophages* that infect viruses themselves.) *Viruses* — infective agents that can only reproduce inside another cell — are pretty simple, but what they cause is not so simple. They may cause no symptoms. They may wreak havoc on us. They may cause something in between or go back and forth.

Virus particles *(virions)* are very small — smaller than we can see with a regular microscope. Yet they still manage to perplex us. Sometimes it even seems like they outwit us. As with any enemy, getting to know what a virus is and how it works is instrumental to thwarting it, and this chapter can help. As you also find out here, some viruses can be prevented by vaccines, while others still evade science's attempts to prevent them.

REMEMBER

There are more viruses than we know out there. As people increase transportation, move into areas with few inhabitants, and have contact with different animals, the world becomes increasingly connected. What may have caused an unknown outbreak in an isolated location that is quickly extinguished can become a large epidemic.

Looking Inside Your Average Virus

TIP

A virus is put together like a burrito. The tortilla is the protein shell. The filling is the genetic instructions, or codes in the form of DNA (deoxyribonucleic acid) or RNA (ribonucleic acid). The DNA strands are often but not always double strands; the RNA is usually but not always single stranded. This genetic code is what lets the virus reprogram and take over a cell.

REMEMBER

Viruses can't do anything on their own. That's why they aren't considered to be alive. They can't make copies of themselves on their own. A virion all by itself isn't enough to make you sick if it can't get inside your cells. Viruses require what living things have in their cells to do what they do best — make copies of themselves. Once a virus is in a living cell, it's almost like it is alive; it will turn that cell into a virus assembly machine.

Successful viruses turn our cells into photocopiers, churning out virions — more and more infectious viral particles. When we get sick, say with the flu, the cells in our bodies may produce as many as 100 trillion virions. That's more than all the stars in the Milky Way.

With all of these copies, there are bound to be mistakes. Viruses make lots of mistakes. They often don't copy their genetic material exactly the same each time. These miscopies are called *mutations.* Not all mutations are bad; many are dead ends. Headlines may say that a virus is mutating, but that's just what viruses do. Viruses mutate; birds fly. Mutations, especially collecting over time, can lead to different variants or strains, and sometimes these changes can evade our immune responses or change how sick they make us.

WARNING

There are many different types — or species — of viruses. Some viruses have round shells; some have long shells. Different viruses use different hooks, or receptors, to hold onto and enter a cell. A specific virus usually only infects a certain species or related species. If your dog gets a cold, you're usually not going to get it. Sometimes, though, a virus can infect different species and can jump from ducks or pigs or bats to us. This jump across species often is another dead end, but sometimes it can lead to a virus that causes us a lot of problems.

Investigating Influenza Viruses

When you say, "I caught the flu," you're often referring to an influenza virus. These are the viruses that cause the sniffles, coughs, achy muscles, fever, and sore throat that can make your life miserable for a week or so. But some influenza viruses — often simply called the flu — can also make you extremely — even deathly — ill. Up to 500 million people are infected by influenza viruses worldwide. In the United States, between 12,000 and 61,000 have died from influenza viruses each year from 2010 through 2020.

Influenza viruses fall into one of four different types — unimaginatively named A, B, C, and D. Influenza viruses can affect many animal species. Some flu viruses just remain in other animals, but some flu subtypes can spread to us from animals, especially farm animals like chickens and pigs. Science has created influenza vaccines against some but not all types. The yearly flu vaccine consists of antigens against type A and type B influenza viruses.

Type A

Type A viruses cause us the most problems. They're the only influenza viruses that have caused a global pandemic, like the COVID-19 pandemic, and they, along with type B, are the types that usually cause seasonal flu outbreaks. (See Chapter 3 for more about COVID-19.)

There are a lot of subtypes of influenza A. There may be 200 main subtypes out there, but only 131 main subtypes have been found. We can't make a vaccine with that many different antigens — all those bits of the virus are needed to create a "Wanted" photo for each subtype. Usually, just a few subtypes dominate any flu season.

So, every year scientists have to make a decision — which two A subtypes and one, or likely two, B subtypes should go into a vaccine. The problem is that it takes a long time to make enough flu vaccines for everyone. Some types of the flu vaccine are grown in chicken eggs, and this takes time. (But don't worry if you're severely allergic to eggs; others are made just in the lab). It takes six months to make a vaccine, so scientists have to pick which subtypes to include half a year ahead of time. They peek at the other side of the globe (Northern or Southern Hemisphere) and figure what's starting to spread, say, in Australia for Northern Hemisphere folks, and what they bet will spread where they are in six months.

REMEMBER

Type A influenza viruses are unusual in that they have tricks to change what they wear, making those immune system "Wanted" photos not always work. They have more tricks for changing the proteins that are on their outside shell, and so they fool our immune system into not knowing who they are. Unlike other types of influenza viruses, Type A has two different ways to change and evade our immune systems. These two ways are called *drift* and *shift*. Influenza A can also infect some animals, and sometimes influenza of animal origins can be a problem for us:

>> *Drift,* also called *antigenic drift,* happens when mutations occur over time. It occurs in all influenza types. After a few mutations, copies of the virus become a bit different from the original viruses. Over time, these small changes build up, and the virus may not even be recognized by our immune system. We can get sick from a subtype that's similar to, but not the same as, one we've seen before. Vaccines continue to work as the virus mutates until there are enough mutations and the antibodies made in response to the vaccine won't recognize the subtype anymore. These slight changes can lead to resistance to drugs we use to treat the flu or even change how this flu subtype affects us.

>> *Shift* occurs only in type A influenza. Influenza A viruses each have two proteins on their surfaces: H (hemagglutinin) and N (neuraminidase). There are 18 different known H's and 11 known N's. That's why there are so many different types of possible influenza A subtypes. These can mix and match — or shift — resulting in big changes in the flu subtype: H1N1, H1N2, H3N2, H7N9. These big changes can result in shifts that leave us unprepared for new subtypes and hence, the risk of flu pandemics.

The following sections go into more detail on two specific Type A viruses: bird flu and swine flu.

Battling bird flu

Birds can get the flu, too. They can get really sick or just a little under the weather, just like us. Sometimes they can pass the flu to us. What makes birds really sick may not make us really sick, but a flu that's nothing for a bird may be catastrophic for us.

Many viruses don't last when they try to infect another species, and even if they infect us, we may not be able to spread the virus to others. But there are specific subtypes that are usually found in birds that, when they cross to humans, can be quite deadly. These subtypes are commonly called *bird flu* or *avian influenza.* Bird flu, though rare, can be fatal. It's fatal for some common types in about half of cases (H5N1 [60 percent], H7N9 [40 percent]). Fortunately, these bird flu subtypes don't have much person-to-person spread.

WARNING

Bird flu usually affects chicken farmers or persons with close contact with these birds. Fortunately, these are rarely transmitted from person to person. If there are outbreaks, farms are closed, culled, and quarantined to prevent further spread. However, bird flu can travel — either between poultry farms or with migratory birds — and different types have been found in many different countries. Our worry is that someday bird flu may spread more easily from person to person.

Suffering from swine flu

H1N1, another type A flu, has been a big worry for us in the past. An H1N1 subtype was the cause of the 1918 influenza pandemic (also called the Spanish flu), which led to the loss of more than 50 million lives worldwide and 650,000 in the United States. This subtype had genes of avian origin, though we haven't yet figured out where it originated.

H1N1 has made news again and more recently caused concern when it began to spread in 2009. The virus crossed over from pigs, which is how it got its name: swine flu. However, H1N1 isn't the only subtype of influenza to originate in pigs; the 2009 version, ultimately dubbed A(H1N1)pdm09, was, however, a new and unique variant not specifically seen before in animals or people, although it was related to prior H1N1 outbreaks.

Swine flu influenza viruses are spread, like other influenza viruses, through droplets in the air or by touching something that, for a graphic example, your pig has sneezed on, and then touching your mouth, nose, or eyes. While the first few cases were found in people who had direct or close contact with pigs, later cases were found to be from person-to-person contact. A vaccine was developed by the end of the year, and the pandemic ended by August 2010, according to the World Health Organization (WHO). In the United States, the CDC estimated there were about 60 million cases and 12,469 deaths from swine flu within the year after it was discovered, with worldwide deaths estimated at around 150,000 to 575,000.

TECHNICAL STUFF

Pigs can have other subtypes of influenza. Subtypes can also mix between birds and pigs before reaching us.

Type B

Type B causes illness similar to Type A. Type B doesn't have subtypes but has two main lineages. It isn't as common a cause of illness as type A is. Generally, type B causes just 25 percent of influenza illnesses during the year. It doesn't change by shift, only by drift, so it doesn't have the same sudden changes that throw off our immune system. Type B also isn't known to infect animals, except for seals, so we don't have to deal with lineages from animals. Type B can still cause serious illness, including pneumonia, and can be fatal in some cases. Vaccines used to include just one B influenza virus, but now most include two.

Type C

Type C usually causes milder illness and is more common in children. Health providers don't vaccinate against Type C and usually don't test for it. You may well have had influenza type C in the past and not recognized it, because symptoms are generally mild. People and some animals are susceptible to this strain of influenza.

Type D

TECHNICAL STUFF

Type D is found mostly in cattle and other animals. It has not been found to cause illness in humans, though some people have antibodies to it, meaning that they've had some exposure to it. There's no vaccination against type D influenza.

Examining Enteroviruses (Including Rhinoviruses)

You've probably had an enterovirus case and didn't even know it. Nine in ten cause no symptoms or just a brief fever without anything remarkable. There are over 80 different types of enteroviruses, and each type has its own footprint. Enteroviruses can cause a common cold; diarrhea; mouth blisters; pink eye; hand, foot, and mouth disease; and even nervous system infections that can lead to paralysis.

These viruses can cause a severe illness in some, a mild illness in others, and just a fever or nothing at all in still others. Enterovirus D68, just to name one, can cause a cold in some, but for some children, it can cause more severe respiratory illness and can leave lasting nerve damage that causes weakness or even paralysis.

There are a few different ways to get sick with an enterovirus:

>> It often spreads when you don't wash your hands frequently, especially after using the toilet.

>> It can spread by fecal-oral transmission, when you get the tiniest amount of stool from someone else in your mouth, often by touching an infected surface and then putting your hand to your mouth.

>> It can spread from having close contact, like shaking hands with someone who hasn't washed their hands well.

>> Directly touching contaminated stool, such as when changing diapers, and then touching your eyes, nose, or mouth can infect you.

>> Contact with fluid from blisters that form in hand, foot, and mouth disease can infect you.

>> Respiratory droplets can spread enteroviruses. Coughing, sneezing, and breathing can create droplets that spread. Any contact with saliva, sputum, eye secretions, or nasal mucus can spread an enterovirus.

>> It can be spread from drinking water with the virus in it, which can occur when tiny amounts of sewage contaminate drinking water, especially where resources are more limited.

WARNING

There's one type of enterovirus that's more worrisome than the rest. Polio is an enterovirus. It causes paralysis in a small number of people who are infected. Usually one in 100 or so infected develop paralysis. Others may just have diarrhea or a fever and not the weakness we worry about. Most people are vaccinated against polio, and the disease has been almost eliminated worldwide. Only one of the three initial types is still spreading, and it's known to be in only a few places.

Rhinoviruses are another viral species in the same family as enterovirus species, and in fact, they are all in the genera enterovirus. They are the most common cause of the cold. They cause many — up to 50 percent — of the sniffles, coughs, and sore throats that we call the common cold. They spread by droplets from coughs, sneezes, and just plain breathing. They can also spread when you touch your face after touching commonly touched items, like doorknobs or countertops.

Usually, rhinoviruses don't cause serious infections, but we'd all rather avoid getting colds. Vaccines haven't been able to help us, though. There are three species (A, B, and C), which include about 160 known types. This means new types keep appearing. So far, scientists haven't been able to come up with a vaccine that creates a response to all of these.

Knowing About Norovirus

There's one virus that everyone notices when it spreads. Norovirus spreads quickly in schools, hospitals, and cruise ships. It spreads mostly by fecal-oral transmission, meaning it spreads when tiny particles from one person's stool (or vomit) get into someone else's mouth. This can happen by direct contact with another person, when food or water is contaminated, or by touching surfaces that someone who is ill has touched. Norovirus can also be aerosolized, spreading in the air to people nearby. This can happen when we flush a toilet or vomit, sending tiny particles into the air that others swallow when they breathe.

It doesn't take much to infect us with norovirus. Our stool can contain billions and billions of virions, but it may take somewhere between ten to 100 of these to infect us. There can be asymptomatic spread.

Infection usually happens fast. We usually get sick 12–48 hours after exposure. Symptoms mostly include vomiting and diarrhea. This can lead to dehydration, along with muscle aches, headaches, and weakness. Usually there isn't much of a fever — if anything there's a low-grade fever. Most people get totally better in two to three days, but norovirus can be serious for folks with other illnesses or who are elderly and can't tolerate the dehydration. A little under 1,000 people are thought to die from norovirus a year in the United States, mostly among the elderly, and over 100,000 need to be hospitalized.

There isn't a vaccine or a specific treatment for norovirus. Rehydration — often with Pedialyte or an oral rehydration serum and sometimes with IV fluids — is what gets us through the dehydration.

Some people are immune to some types of norovirus thanks to a gene (FUT2) that they are born with. But this works against only some genotypes of norovirus. There are ten main groups and at least 48 different genotypes.

Others develop immunity to specific types after getting sick, but not to all the genotypes, and it's not clear how long this immunity lasts.

Understanding HIV

Human immunodeficiency virus, or HIV, is responsible for more deaths than any other virus in recent history. Over 75 million people have been infected and about 33 million have died since the epidemic was first recognized. The first cases of AIDS (Acquired Immune Deficiency Syndrome) were identified in 1981, and the virus was identified in 1983.

Because of fear of the virus, stigma, denial, and discrimination developed toward those who were infected, thought to be infected, or in high-risk groups. Many have worked to combat these issues.

HIV can weaken the immune system and make us more prone to other infections we would otherwise fight off without ever getting sick. The virus attacks the immune system, and if not treated, it will go on to cause AIDS, where these opportunistic infections that we normally can fight off make us sick. About half of those with HIV develop AIDS in eight to ten years without treatment.

It's possible to have HIV without symptoms for many years. Some people have initial flu-like symptoms (fever, fatigue, rash, night sweats, muscle aches, sore throat, swollen lymph nodes) about two to four weeks after the initial infection. These symptoms can be overlooked because they seem like many other viruses (commonly mistaken for "mono" or Epstein-Barr virus, or EBV, in particular).

There's no vaccine against HIV; however, there are many ways to reduce our chance of developing HIV. Safer sex, including using condoms when appropriate, has reduced sexual transmission risks. Using clean needles for any injection, including injection drugs, reduces transmission.

There are also medications, called *antiretrovirals*, that can reduce transmission. Without treatment, 15 percent to 45 percent of mothers used to pass HIV onto their babies during pregnancy, at birth, or by breastfeeding. Treatment given at birth reduced this risk. Now, treatment for the mother before, during, and after pregnancy greatly reduces the risk of transmission and lets HIV-positive mothers breastfeed.

These same antiretrovirals can help prevent transmission to us. Those who are at high risk for HIV, through sex or injection drug use, can take a daily pill to reduce their risk. This is called PrEP, or pre-exposure prophylaxis. This reduces but does not entirely eliminate the risk of infection.

Another preventive measure is PEP — or post-exposure prophylaxis — which can be taken after a specific exposure, such as through sex, an injection, a needlestick, or other health-worker exposure. This reduces but does not entirely eliminate the risk of infection. These antiretrovirals are best taken within the first 24 hours after exposure but must be taken at least in the first 72 hours. The medications need to be taken daily for four weeks and then stopped.

These same medications that are used to prevent HIV transmission also treat HIV. Treatments developed in the last few decades mean that with treatment, you can live as long with HIV as without it. These medications do not cure HIV. They keep HIV in check, but if these medications are stopped, HIV can bounce back. Medications need to be taken as prescribed, usually daily; otherwise, resistance can develop and the medications may not work anymore for that person. Nearly 20 million people with HIV currently take antiretroviral drugs to manage this disease. Treatment is prevention. Those who take these medications and have the virus fully suppressed won't transmit the virus to others.

Trying to Say Goodbye to Measles

Measles, once a common, extremely contagious, but sometimes deadly illness in children, is a viral disease we're trying to say goodbye to. It's a virus that causes a high fever, runny nose, cough, and pink eye. It may just seem like a bad cold at first, but then three to five days later, the rash it's known for pops up.

We don't have a drug that cures measles, but most people get better in one to two weeks. About one in five need to be hospitalized. Some people develop lung or brain infections. Between one and three in every 1,000 infected will die. Measles also weakens the immune system for a bit, so you may get sick from another infection even after getting better. In rare cases, years after getting better, a fatal brain disease develops out of the blue in those who have recovered from measles.

WARNING

The problem is that measles spreads silently in the air, and it spreads far. It can drift and infect people far away in a sports stadium, who never even saw the person who was ill. It can also spread before the telltale rash appears. One person can cause 12, maybe 18, new infections if no one is vaccinated. It also doesn't make people sick for another 10 to 12 days, so it can be hard to track where they got it.

Before there was a vaccine, 2 to 3 million people, mostly children, died each year from measles. With vaccination, we have been able to eliminate chains of transmission in many countries. Measles was declared eliminated in the United States in 2000, but cases pop up each year, often a souvenir from travel possibly followed by local spread. Worldwide, too many people still die from it, around 200,000 a year.

REMEMBER

Because measles is so easily transmitted, you need almost everyone to be in this together to say goodbye to measles. The virus is really good at spreading to a lot of people, invisibly, all at once. Because it can spread so easily, at least 19 out of every 20 people need to be vaccinated to eliminate measles altogether. Where there has been a reluctance to vaccinate, the measles takes advantage and hides out, causing outbreaks to pop up, mostly among the unvaccinated.

Measles is different from German measles (also called rubella), which has now been eliminated from the Western Hemisphere and is on the decline elsewhere.

Checking Out the Cause of Chicken Pox: Varicella

The varicella virus causes chicken pox. Chicken pox used to be a common infection in children, until vaccination for chicken pox made it uncommon in the United States. In the United Kingdom and other countries, vaccination isn't routine, so cases are more common.

This virus is most common in children, but more worrisome in adults and especially pregnant women. About 1 in 5,000 infected adults die from chicken pox, but many more adults need to be hospitalized. It is worse in those with weakened immune systems. If most people are vaccinated but a few are not, the average age of infected people grows older. Those few may not come in contact with the virus early on when they are kids, but instead it may take years for them to be infected and they get sick as adults, when the disease is more serious. This can be a problem, and it's important to be vaccinated.

Varicella looks a lot like measles. Its rash starts first on the abdomen and then spreads. The measles rash starts first on the forehead and face and then spreads. The measles rash is mostly flat, but chicken pox has raised bumps with liquid inside, which become itchy. Both can spread in the air. Both can infect many people quickly if others aren't immune.

TIP

This virus remains in our bodies after we get better. It can stay dormant, or asleep, in our nerves. It can then return many years later as a painful rash in just a small patch on just one side of the body. This is *shingles* (or herpes zoster), and it only develops in people who have had chicken pox when the virus awakens in one *dermatome* (or area of skin with nerves coming from one spinal nerve root). Shingles can recur multiple times. If you've had chicken pox in the past, the shingles vaccine can prevent this painful disease from affecting you.

Fighting Ebola

Ebola wasn't known about until 1976. In that year it suddenly caused separate outbreaks in the now Democratic Republic of the Congo and South Sudan. It's a virus that remains most of the time in bats, largely in Central and Western Africa, but every once in a while, it spreads to humans. It can spread from contact with a bat or from hunting or picking up another animal that's sick or dead from Ebola.

WARNING

Ebola is something we consider important to control because it can kill about half of those infected and can close down many hospitals and clinics, resulting in others not being able to get care.

The virus spreads by direct contact with blood or other body fluids (such as vomit, diarrhea, urine, breast milk, sweat, and semen) as well as bedsheets or clothing contaminated by the body fluids of an infected person. The virus often spreads in hospitals when people who are sick seek care, especially women in labor as it can cause more bleeding in labor.

Ebola develops 2 to 21 days after exposure (usually 8 to 10 days). Ebola doesn't spread before symptoms. There are usually two stages of Ebola:

» **Dry stage:** The first stage is the dry stage, characterized by fever, aches and pains, sore throat, and fatigue. This stage can be mistaken for influenza or the flu. Some people also have hiccups, which can help identify the illness as Ebola because hiccups and fever are not that common.

» **Wet stage:** The disease then progresses to the wet stage (with more fevers and now diarrhea and vomiting and sometimes bleeding and miscarriage in pregnant women). It is in the wet stage that people are very sick and often become confused. They need the help of others to take care of them, and they are also the most infectious then. Ebola can spread from the diarrhea, sweat, and other body fluids, making others sick. The virus often infects family members who care for those who are sick, nurses and doctors, and those involved in preparing for funerals as bodies after death remain infectious.

Some people have very mild cases, and others have very serious cases. The initial amount of virus someone has in their blood when tested can predict their chance of getting better. People who get better from Ebola can go back to their regular lives and aren't infectious once they clear the virus. However, the virus can hide where the immune system doesn't notice the virus as quickly. For example, the virus can remain in men's testes and result in spreading the virus through sex, even a year later. Some people also can have eye symptoms and vision loss later on because the virus can remain in the eye and cause inflammation.

Most outbreaks have been fewer than 100 cases. It wasn't until Ebola was identified in West Africa in 2014, as it spread largely between Liberia, Sierra Leone, and Guinea, that we ever saw a large epidemic over a few hundred. This outbreak spread unnoticed at first but then rapidly caused over 28,000 cases and over 11,000 deaths. A large international commitment of people working in collaboration was required to control it, as the virus often spreads among clinics and hospitals, affecting those most needed to fight it and making it even harder to contain.

Ebola is called a *viral hemorrhagic fever* (VHF). That means it is a virus that causes a fever, which can be accompanied by bleeding, often with a severe infection affecting multiple organs. There's often a lot of fear around the bleeding, but in reality bleeding is not that common and usually not the worrisome part of the disease. Instead, it's that the virus can affect multiple organs, making it difficult for them to function together.

We're on the lookout for other related and unrelated viruses that also cause VHFs. These include Lassa (a close relative to Ebola), yellow fever, dengue (rarely causes a VHF), Crimean-Congo hemorrhagic fever, Rift Valley fever, and about ten others. We never want to have a case of a viral hemorrhagic fever, but although these viruses can seem scary, if the correct actions are taken to stop transmission and control the outbreak, they can be stopped.

Surveying Variola (Smallpox)

Smallpox is the only human virus that humans have ever eradicated. There were two different variants. The more dangerous version would kill 30 percent of those infected and leave survivors with scars, frequently on their faces.

This virus led to the first inoculations with bits of material from smallpox skin lesions. These date back to at least the tenth century BC in China. The virus was so bad that it seemed better to be injected with a small amount and have a mild infection with some risk than to have a severe infection later with greater risk of dying. It also inspired the first vaccine, using cowpox to create a mild infection that protected against smallpox in 1796. (See Chapter 5 for more on the development of the smallpox vaccine.)

The World Health Organization, a little under 200 years later, building on the success of the vaccine, led a large campaign to vaccinate and track down every last case until they finally succeeded in 1977. In the last 100 years before it was eradicated, variola is thought to have killed 500 million people. There was one last death from smallpox after it had been eradicated, a visitor to a laboratory where it was still studied. After this occurred, stocks of smallpox virus were destroyed around the world. Only the United States and Russia are known to have kept stocks in laboratories.

The upper arms of those who were vaccinated for smallpox have a small scar that shows they were vaccinated. Vaccination was stopped in 1972 in the United States, after the disease was eliminated from the United States. By 1980, vaccination had stopped worldwide. It just wasn't needed anymore, but some people, those who work in labs with the virus or military personnel, may still be vaccinated because there is concern about bioterrorism from this virus.

Chapter **3**

The Crowned Virus: Coronavirus

COVID-19 seemed to appear out of the blue and suddenly, the term "coronavirus" dominated the news. We knew nothing about COVID-19 before it appeared at the end of 2019, but we did know a thing or two about other coronaviruses and respiratory viruses. Not all coronaviruses are deadly; in fact, you've probably had a coronavirus many times in your life. Coronaviruses cause many cases of the common cold. But on the flip side, they can also cause some unusual and deadly outbreaks, as the COVID-19 pandemic has shown.

Vaccines are the final ticket out of the current COVID-19 pandemic. Fortunately, scientists had discovered from past coronaviruses and already had terrific ideas about how to make effective vaccines. Building on past work, effective and fully tested vaccines hit the market within one year. But vaccines work only if people are willing to take them. It's vaccinations, not vaccines, that save lives.

In this chapter, we review the different types of coronaviruses and discuss the serious and not-so-serious coronavirus outbreaks that have occurred. Lastly, we dig into the details of how COVID-19 shut down numerous countries, check out symptoms, explore the search for treatments, and explain the development of the vaccines with the potential to stop transmission in its tracks.

Identifying the Coronavirus in Humans

The first person to ever see a human coronavirus and snap a photo was June Almeida in 1964. Growing up poor in Glasgow, Scotland, she didn't seem primed to find something that would shape so many lives. Her brother died from an infectious disease (diphtheria) as a child, and she dropped out of school at 16 to earn money and found work in laboratories. She developed her own techniques to find and photograph the tiniest virus particles, otherwise lost under cells and debris under a microscope.

The Common Cold Unit team in Great Britain had a swab from one boy with a cold that seemed totally different from anything they'd seen. They did all sorts of lab studies but just couldn't find it under the microscope. Dr. David Tyrell at the Common Cold Unit had heard that Almeida could find what others could not.

Their hunch that Almeida could help paid off. These virus particles looked different, covered with spikes, forming what looked like a hazy halo. Almeida called this a coronavirus, since "corona" means crown in Latin. Almeida knew she'd seen this before in samples from mice and chickens. Sure enough, the virus strains she remembered were other coronavirus strains. The first coronavirus had actually been identified decades earlier, but not named, in sick baby chicks who had "colds" that turned deadly in the 1930s. Fortunately, these coronaviruses don't usually crossover from animals to make humans sick.

When Almeida tried to then publish these photos, they were initially rejected. "They're just bad photos of the flu virus," she was told. From their first sighting, coronaviruses have been confused with the flu, but Almeida was right: Coronaviruses are unique. The name, in fact, seemed to be a bit of a premonition about how important they would become.

For her work on coronaviruses and other viruses, she would be given a doctorate of science, making her Dr. June Almeida.

Meanwhile, across the Atlantic at the same time, another researcher, Dr. Dorothy Hamre, was busy studying a virus in Chicago with colleagues when she also found another strain of coronavirus from a medical student with a cold. Scientists would go on to find hundreds of coronaviruses, mostly in other mammals and birds.

REMEMBER

Initially, four human coronavirus species were identified; all caused common colds. It wouldn't be until 2002 that coronaviruses became known for anything more than colds. And over the following 20 years, coronaviruses would show themselves to cause much more.

NAMING THE COLD AND OTHER VIRUSES

There's not just one sort of cold. A whole bunch of viruses cause colds. Some have some interesting names. For example:

- The coronavirus has a regal name. *Corona* means "crown" in Latin, as in coronation. It was actually named for the solar corona, or the halo of light surrounding the sun. All those spikes looked a bit like a fuzzy halo.

- The rhinovirus and the rhino are named for the same thing — the nose. The rhino's big horn and the rhinovirus, which affects our noses, come from the Greek for "nose."

- The flu is just a nickname for influenza, which comes from the Italian for "influence." Outbreaks seemed like forces of nature, influenced by the stars.

- Some names just reflect where the virus is found in people. Adenovirus, for example, is named because it was first isolated from the adenoids, the immune system glands in the back of the throat with the tonsils. Enterovirus is named because it passes through our intestines (*entero-* meaning "intestinal").

In 2002, SARS (severe acute respiratory syndrome) appeared in southern China and would cause a worldwide epidemic of respiratory illness with over 8,000 known cases, leading to death in one in ten of those infected. In 2012, MERS (Middle East respiratory syndrome) was found in Saudi Arabia, which caused fewer than 1,000 cases but deaths in over a third of those known infected. (We cover SARS and MERS in more detail later in this chapter.)

Then along came SARS–CoV–2, causing a worldwide pandemic of COVID-19, beginning in late 2019 and causing over 1.8 million deaths and 84 million known cases in 2020. We discuss COVID-19 in greater detail later in this chapter.

Combatting the Common Cold Coronavirus

If you're old enough to read this, you've almost certainly had a coronavirus that wasn't COVID. Four types of coronaviruses cause regular old colds in people. People usually have one to three colds a year. About one in ten of these colds were probably from a coronavirus. During some coronavirus outbreaks, up to three in ten colds have been from coronaviruses.

Animals, even domestic animals, also get coronaviruses. Coronaviruses can affect cats and dogs, even parakeets, ferrets, and mice. Usually these don't spread between different animal species, but there are occasions when the virus has jumped species.

In the following sections, we define colds and their causes — including coronaviruses — and explain when a cold isn't actually a cold.

What is a cold, exactly?

REMEMBER

Colds are upper respiratory tract infections. That means the virus gets into your nose and/or throat and gives you the sniffles and makes you sneeze. Symptoms can vary among people and viruses, but colds generally include some of these symptoms:

>> Runny or stuffy nose

>> Sneezing

>> Sore throat

>> Feeling congested

>> Cough

>> Mild body aches

>> Feeling warm, but not having a high temperature

>> Just feeling "under the weather"

You may have a discharge from your nose that becomes thicker or yellower, but this doesn't mean the infection that's bugging us is more serious than a cold.

Most people get better in a week to ten days. Children under 5 are more likely to get colds because they haven't experienced as many colds before and may not have immunity to the colds circulating.

WARNING

Cold viruses that may make some people just have the sniffles can make others, especially the very young, the old, or the immunocompromised, become sicker with the virus. Always see your health provider if a cold becomes worse, causing a fever, difficulty breathing, or other more serious symptoms.

What causes a cold?

Colds are caused by viruses, but no one virus is responsible. Well over 100 different viruses cause common colds. That's the problem with finding a cure or vaccine for colds; there are just too many different types. You usually won't know which type of cold virus you have, although certain symptoms or the time of year can give you an idea:

>> **Rhinoviruses:** If you have a cold, it's most likely a rhinovirus. About 80 percent of colds are caused by rhinoviruses. There are over 160 different types of rhinoviruses, meaning your immune system may not recognize all of them. These colds can occur at any time of the year, peaking in spring and autumn.

>> **Coronaviruses:** These cause about 10 percent of common colds, most commonly in the winter and early spring.

>> **RSV (respiratory syncytial virus)** season begins in the fall and continues into the spring, causing colds for most of us. RSV can make babies and small children very sick.

>> **Human metapnuemoviruses** also spread at the same time as RSV and infect almost every young child, but can still cause reinfection later in life.

>> **Enteroviruses** commonly cause summer colds.

>> **Adenoviruses** can spread year round but especially in winter and spring. They can cause pink eye with cold symptoms.

>> **Parainfluenza** comes in four different types and is more common in spring, summer, and fall.

>> **Coxsackieviruses** spread more in the summer and autumn and can also cause hand, foot, and mouth disease (a rash in the mouth and on the hands).

REMEMBER

Fewer colds occurred during the COVID-19 outbreak. Social distancing, hand-washing, masks, and limited travel helped squash them. The problem is that cold outbreaks will just bounce back when we stop trying to control COVID-19. A lot of children haven't had the colds they usually would have had due to decreased exposure. Many will be vulnerable once life is back to normal and will spread these colds.

When is a cold not a cold?

Not all "colds" are actually colds. Some illnesses that have similar symptoms to colds actually belong in other categories, as you find out in the following sections. It's important to recognize the differences, because while time is the best cure for colds, other diseases may require specific treatments to prevent more serious problems. Some viruses are fine for most of us but can be really dangerous for others.

Recognizing RSV (respiratory syncytial virus)

Most of us get the virus RSV again and again. It's "just a cold," and we feel better soon. Illnesses depend not just on the virus that causes them but on the person who gets sick. What is a cold for us may be a deadly lung infection for babies. This is true for RSV in particular. For little babies and toddlers, it can mean a trip to the hospital. In small babies (under 6 months), about one in every 50 to 100 infected need to be hospitalized. They may have coughing, wheezing, and problems breathing. Some elderly adults and those with immune system problems also can become pretty sick from RSV, as well as other common cold viruses. Worldwide, around 160,000 people die each year from RSV, most of them small children.

There's currently no vaccine against RSV, although scientists continue to work on developing one.

Fighting the flu

Whoever said "it's just the flu" had a cold and not the flu. The flu can feel terrible. It can make you feel like you just got hit by a truck.

The flu can cause that same stuffy nose, sneezing, and cough that the common cold does. And you may just have mild symptoms. But for most of us, the flu is no cold. The flu can come with a sudden high fever, a deep cough, muscle aches, chills, and exhaustion. There's much less sneezing and fewer stuffy noses and a lot more body aches and lung symptoms.

Each year, around the world, it's estimated that one-quarter to one-half of a million people die from the flu. One in ten people get the flu each year on average in the United States, although this can vary from year to year. Deaths in the United States from the flu range from 12,000 to 61,000 people each year, many of whom are elderly. Influenza can also be pretty severe for children. In the United States, around 100 children die each year from the flu; half of these have no other health issues.

REMEMBER

The flu vaccine can help reduce your chance of getting the flu as well as its severity if you do. If you do get the flu, you can ask your health provider about getting a medication for it. This sort of med won't make the flu go away but will reduce how long it lasts. Talk to your healthcare provider about the risks and benefits. See Chapter 6 for details on the flu vaccine.

Hearing about whooping cough

Whooping cough, also called pertussis, sounds just like that — a whoop. It's a bit like a barking seal. But it starts just like a cold for the first week or two. For most people, it just causes a runny nose, maybe a low-grade fever, and an occasional, mild cough. But after the first week or two, the cough gets worse, becoming a barking seal cough. Fits of coughing can be exhausting and may even be followed by vomiting. It can last for many weeks.

REMEMBER

This can all be prevented with the pertussis vaccine, which is given with some tetanus vaccines: Tdap in adults and DTaP for kids (the *ap/aP* stands for acellular pertussis; Chapters 8 and 9 go into more detail on these vaccines). It's important to be vaccinated, even if not for ourselves. Whooping cough is an annoyance for most of us, but it can be a deadly infection for tiny babies. It's important everyone — grandma, uncle, cousin — is vaccinated for pertussis when they go to visit a new baby.

Specific antibiotics can help reduce the symptoms and the risk of spreading the disease if diagnosed early, as only certain antibiotics work and these work only in the first few weeks.

Suffering through strep throat

Most sore throats accompany ordinary cold viruses, but sometimes they may be due to a type of bacteria called group A Streptococcus (group A strep). In general, about three in ten children with a sore throat have strep throat. In comparison, just one in ten adults with a sore throat have strep. A rapid test or a culture can confirm whether someone has strep. Some folks carry the bacteria without symptoms; when they get sick from a virus, they may test positive for strep throat and it's hard to tell what is causing it.

Your sore throat may be due to strep if you have

>> Fever

>> White patches in the back of the throat

>> Tender lymph nodes in the neck

>> No cough

The more symptoms you have, the more likely you have strep throat; however, even with all four symptoms, only about half of adults have strep throat. Most sore throats are just viruses.

Most cases of strep throat occur in children, often between ages 5 and 15. Parents of children and those who work with children (such as day-care workers and teachers) are also more at risk. Anyone who has had recent contact with someone with strep throat (for example, at home or in a dorm) is also at increased risk.

You want to identify and treat strep throat, especially in children, as it can cause rare but serious side effects, such as rheumatic fever (which can cause heart, joint, and brain problems) or kidney damage. Antibiotics can prevent this. The antibiotics can also help treat the sore throat and prevent transmission to others.

Sore throats can sometimes be more complicated, even if it's not strep. If your tonsils in the back of your throat look particularly big, you have any difficulty swallowing, or your neck is swelling or you find it difficult to move your neck, it's important to be seen by a healthcare professional. You may have inflammation of your tonsils (*tonsilitis*) or even an *abscess* (a collection of pus forming) or a more serious infection of your neck.

Warding off superinfections

When you get a common cold, you may want to know whether antibiotics would help. When it's just a cold, the answer is no. That's because colds are caused by viruses and not bacteria. Antibiotics only work against bacteria. We don't have antivirals for the common cold. We only have treatments for symptoms (fever, sore throat, sneezing, cough, aches).

Taking antibiotics when you have a virus means having all the risks and no benefit. Antibiotics can cause side effects such as allergic reactions, rashes, and dangerous diarrhea. They can also cause bacteria harmlessly found on your skin, in your nose, or in your intestines to become resistant. If you do develop an infection in the future, the antibiotic may no longer work against the bacteria.

But when you're sick, there's often still that nagging worry that a cold can turn into a more serious infection, and that antibiotics may help ward off complications. A change in mucus color, for example, causes many people concern. But if you first start blowing your nose and it's clear, but after a few days the mucus gets thicker and yellower and then maybe greenish or grayish-greenish, this actually isn't a sign of bacteria. It's just a sign of your immune cells showing up to fight.

But there are times when a cold can lead to a bacterial infection. These are called *superinfections* — when bacteria infects us on top of a virus. Sometimes all that congestion can lead to inflammation and then even a bacterial infection in your sinuses, or *sinusitis*. Sinus infections include many of the common cold symptoms — runny or stuffy nose, cough, sore throat — but may also include face pain or pressure, postnasal drip (dripping down the back of your throat), and new bad breath.

Not all sinusitis needs antibiotics, as it isn't always due to bacteria. At first, it's usually still due to the virus and the inflammation your immune system creates. Over time, though, bacteria can grow in the fluid and inflammation that have built up.

Do talk to your healthcare provider if you have

>> Sinusitis for ten days without improvement

>> Symptoms now worsening after initially improving

>> Severe headache or facial pain

>> Fever, especially if it lasts for three to four days

Also talk to your provider if you're immunocompromised or have poorly controlled diabetes.

USING THE COMMON COLD AS A CANCER CURE

Colds may just have their uses. They can be a medical tool. It may seem counterintuitive, but colds can be a futuristic medical delivery service.

Cold viruses target certain cells, enter them, and then don't make us that sick. It may be possible to tweak them a bit and harness them to act as carrier pigeons, carrying the directions for treatments or vaccines where we need it in our bodies, without causing any additional problems.

This is something scientists have been thinking about. One common cold virus — adenovirus — has been used to target and destroy cancer cells. Certain modifications ensure the virus targets just one type of cell, leaving the rest of our cells nice and healthy.

These same adenoviruses have been used as vaccine pack ponies. They carry the genetic instructions to build the antigen for certain vaccines, including those for COVID-19 and Ebola. These viruses are adjusted in the lab to keep them from replicating (making copies of themselves) so they won't make you sick and won't spread to anyone else.

Usually we want to have antibodies and immunity to a virus, but here we actually don't. We don't want our own immune systems to foil our plans and attack and stop the cold virus before it reaches its destination. To avoid this, strains are used that we don't commonly see, even if we do see other strains of the same virus. Other viruses that are much less common than a cold virus are often used, such as viruses or strains seen only in animals.

Colds can lead to ear infections, especially in children. Sometimes a cold can cause fluid build-up in the middle ear (behind your eardrums). If your eustachian tubes aren't draining the fluid out well from your middle ear down to the upper throat, you can end up with bacteria swimming in that fluid. Because viruses can also cause ear infections, many pediatricians will watch to see whether symptoms improve in two to three days before prescribing antibiotics.

REMEMBER

Do contact your provider right away if you or your child have

>> Hearing loss

>> Pus or fluid coming from the ear

>> Fever

>> Worsening symptoms

>> Pain lasting at least two to three days

Surveying SARS and MERS

COVID-19 wasn't the first coronavirus on the block. It wasn't even the first one to cause a deadly disease that spread from country to country. SARS-CoV-2, the virus that causes COVID-19, is actually the third deadly coronavirus to appear in the last 20 years. The following sections discuss the first two: SARS and MERS.

Severe acute respiratory syndrome (SARS)

Coronaviruses went suddenly from being only typical colds to having a deadly reputation in 2003.

In southern China in late 2002, a man died from what seemed like a terrible flu. Then there were more cases. It spread mostly through droplets via close contact but occasionally via aerosols that stayed in the air longer and traveled farther. The time from exposure to the onset of symptoms ranged from one to 14 days, with four to six days being the norm. Fortunately, transmission seemed to occur only from those with symptoms, which included muscle aches, fevers, sore throats, and serious lung problems. The outbreak spread in hospitals to other patients and to healthcare workers in different countries from Vietnam to Canada, eventually affecting 30 countries.

Delays in reporting gave the virus time to spread. Some doctors tried to sound the alarm that this virus was something very different and should be taken seriously.

More than 10 percent of those affected died. The elderly were more likely to get severely ill; over half of those over 65 died. Overall, 8,000 people became sick, and 774 died. In the United States, no deaths were reported, although some returning travelers were affected. Fortunately, the epidemic was contained almost entirely in 2003. The last cases known were in 2004, related to lab accidents, but were not found to spread further.

REMEMBER

SARS (severe acute respiratory syndrome, or SARS-CoV-1) showed scientists the importance of timely reporting of cases of novel and dangerous infectious diseases. The world found out how important it was to work together to stop diseases spreading rapidly between countries. It became clear how important it was to be open and honest about cases so that everyone could work together. The SARS virus had close relatives among bats and even closer ones among palm civets (furry animals that look like cats but actually aren't). Other deadly viruses exist in animals, including other coronaviruses, that can make an appearance in humans.

No vaccine for SARS is currently available and tested, but possible vaccines were developed during the virus's spread. However, when the outbreak stopped, there were no cases to prevent in order to test for efficacy.

Middle East respiratory syndrome (MERS)

Middle East respiratory syndrome, or MERS, another disease caused by a coronavirus, also caused deadly outbreaks. In 2012, a man in Saudi Arabia became ill. Other cases soon followed. Cases tended to be in Saudi Arabia or neighboring countries, hence the name Middle East respiratory syndrome. Nurses, doctors, and caregivers of the sick often became ill. Cough and fever often progressed to pneumonia, needing intubation and machines to breathe, and kidney failure, requiring dialysis.

MERS (technically known as MERS-CoV) was deadlier than SARS. At first, almost one in two diagnosed would die. Later, after medical teams became more experienced at treating patients, almost two out of three would survive.

The virus spread with travel. It showed up in London and in Indiana. It arrived in South Korea in 2015 via a traveler, causing just under 200 cases and under 40 deaths.

It continues to spread year after year, but in the first decade of its spread, it was diagnosed in only a few hundred a year, not more than 500.

Unlike other coronaviruses, where the animal source sometimes isn't clear, this one was tied to a very clear source: camels. This virus seemed to come from bats originally, but then spread among camels, especially baby ones. People working with camels were more likely to be infected, but it can also spread from person to person, though fortunately it didn't cause very large outbreaks. Although outbreaks are not as large as COVID-19 or even SARS, each case of MERS is deadlier, and it continues to reappear year after year.

REMEMBER

MERS currently lacks a vaccine, but research for vaccines for MERS and SARS (see the preceding section) helped scientists develop the COVID-19 vaccines so quickly. Researchers built on the work they were already doing on coronaviruses and thus were able to develop effective vaccines more quickly than they could have from scratch.

COVID-19: The Novel (and Specially Confounding) Coronavirus

2020 became the year of the COVID-19 pandemic. The virus, technically named SARS-CoV-2, spread to every continent and seemingly every country after starting in Wuhan, China. Cases quickly overwhelmed hospitals around the globe — northern Italy, Iran, New York City, and then other cities, states, and countries, until almost every country reported cases.

The following sections trace the history of COVID-19, from its detection to the development of vaccines and beyond.

Reviewing the start of the pandemic

The official name the World Health Organization (WHO) gave to the disease caused by SARS-CoV-2 is *COVID-19* ("Coronavirus Disease 2019"). It isn't entirely clear from which animal the new coronavirus was first transmitted to humans in the Chinese city of Wuhan, a city with over a million inhabitants. It probably originated from bats. It was also found that pangolin (scaly anteaters that are an endangered species, protected by international law, but sometimes eaten illegally) carry similar viruses, but data has shown this is not the ancestor of the SARS-CoV-2 that has been spreading among us.

The first COVID-19 case in the United States was reported on January 19, 2020. A 35-year-old man showed up at an urgent care clinic in Snohomish County, Washington, complaining of a persistent dry cough. He volunteered the information that he had recently visited family in Wuhan, China. A month later, an outbreak causing 35 deaths was identified in a nursing home, having spread there by silent community transmission. The virus was spreading, undetected.

Testing was limited and often unavailable. Accurate tests were limited in number. By March 17, 2020, COVID-19 was present in all 50 of the United States.

On March 11, 2020, the WHO characterized the COVID-19 outbreak as a pandemic. A *pandemic* is a global outbreak of disease. Because there was little to no preexisting immunity against the new virus, it spread worldwide.

This virus seemed to close the world. Suddenly, wild animals walked on once-busy streets and the Himalayas were visible where they hadn't been seen in decades due to pollution. Families watched on cellphones, unable to be at the bedside, as their loved ones struggled to survive and sometimes died in hospitals.

Exhausted healthcare workers tried to keep so many sick patients alive, without enough protective equipment and supplies. Healthcare personnel found ways to respond to surges and to care for patients on the fly. Public health officials found ways to prevent surges by advising limited mixing, avoiding close social contact, and using masks. Scientists started to build on what had been learned from past outbreaks — whether of different coronaviruses, flu viruses, or even outbreaks like Ebola and polio — and apply possible solutions to this new disease.

REMEMBER

By the end of 2020, 1.8 million deaths had been reported to the World Health Organization and many more were thought to be undercounted. Some who survived have had symptoms that persisted, making it hard to breathe or carry on their regular lives. The elderly population has been particularly hard-hit by this virus, but no one is immune (though children seem to be the least susceptible to it). People with existing health conditions, most especially Down syndrome (likely due to a gene on the extra chromosome) as well as diabetes, sickle cell disease, hypertension, lung diseases, cancer, or obesity, have been shown to be even more vulnerable.

The virus spread in waves, affecting some countries, then others, and then returning to countries that had started to get back to normal. It spread before people even knew they had it. Ramping up testing to track the virus took a lot of work; initially the virus spread while testing was delayed. Even well-resourced hospitals struggled with surging numbers of patients. It was hard to find enough staff and supplies for intensive care, let alone enough oxygen, in some settings.

Countries around the world went into lockdown and cut off travel. Without a cure or a vaccine, we had to find ways to control this virus. It was a bit like learning to fly a plane after taking off.

At first, medical personnel relied on non-pharmaceutical interventions (NPIs) to prevent spread and keep hospitals from being overwhelmed. People were asked not to gather in large groups and to stand at least 2 meters or so (6 feet) apart. As we discovered more about the virus, people were asked to wear masks to prevent silently spreading the virus to others. Handwashing and good hygiene are always very important, but initially this pandemic prompted a lot of cleaning — even of mail and groceries — that we eventually realized wasn't necessary. Over time, it became clear that direct contact with surfaces didn't play a major role in the spread of the virus as it does with many cold viruses.

Instead, the virus spread mostly through the air, usually to those closest, but sometimes as aerosols further away. Businesses set up temperature checks for people entering stores and work, although studies showed that many people didn't run fevers with this illness, so temperature checks weren't preventing much transmission. Learning on the fly, finding the best solutions, and then constantly updating information helped prevent transmission.

Charting the course of the infection

The COVID pathogen, SARS-CoV-2, infects the upper and lower respiratory tracts. After an incubation period of five to six (up to a maximum of 14) days, it causes flu-like symptoms, such as a general malaise, headache, dry cough, fever, chills, and diarrhea. In some cases, the initially mild disease can become extremely severe, leading to pneumonia and even acute lung failure.

The following sections discuss initial symptoms, hospitalization risks, and the phenomenon of long COVID.

Initial symptoms

WARNING

What's been so tricky about stopping COVID-19 is that, as with some other illnesses, you can spread the virus when you feel fine. The virus, like many others, is most infectious right before and after symptoms begin. These symptoms at first are very mild and easy to ignore. Infections that require isolating and quarantine can lead to denial of the risk since you feel perfectly fine. Early symptoms mimic those of dozens of illnesses, making it easier to deny that you may have COVID-19.

When symptoms start, you may have any or all of the following:

>> Fever

>> Headache

>> Sore throat

>> Fatigue

>> Congestion

>> Cough

>> Loss of sense of smell, even without a stuffy nose

Symptoms usually start out mild and may stay that way. Some people have few or no symptoms for the whole course of the illness. Others, often by day eight or so, have difficulty breathing. Some may have low oxygen levels and just feel fatigued. Others may have abdominal pain or other symptoms.

All these symptoms *can* occur, but they don't necessarily *have to.*

REMEMBER

Risks for hospitalization

Most who develop COVID-19 don't need hospitalization, but any chronic condition can increase your risk of serious illness. To name just a few, you have a higher risk of serious illness and hospitalization if you

WARNING

>> Are elderly (the highest risk factor; 80 percent of deaths occur in those over age 65)

>> Are overweight, especially if you fall into the obese category

>> Have high blood pressure

>> Are diabetic

>> Have sickle cell anemia

>> Have Down syndrome

>> Are pregnant

People of color have been at higher risk for COVID-19 and more have died in the United States.

Of those who are hospitalized, around 25 percent require critical care, including possibly mechanical ventilation or dialysis. Crowded ICUs and short staffing can increase the risk of patients dying.

It's not always easy to guess who will get seriously sick. Adults in their 20s and 30s, as well as some children, with no clear health risks, can require hospitalization. Many tragic deaths have occurred among those much younger. Those who work essential jobs, whether in grocery stores or food production, have faced higher rates of illness in the United States.

When the virus first hit, there weren't any specific treatments for COVID-19. Through careful study of patients enrolled in trials, it was found that steroid treatment in those needing oxygen reduced the chance of dying. Most other treatments didn't reduce the chance of death, but some were found to help people get better more quickly.

Long COVID

REMEMBER

Of those who get better, some have lingering symptoms, whether they were in the hospital or not. They may feel like the infection never fully goes away. This condition, known as *long COVID*, can affect anyone who has had the virus, even those who never had symptoms. Long COVID can cause

>> Lasting fatigue

>> Difficulty thinking clearly, or "brain fog"

>> Continuing loss of taste or smell

>> Breathing difficulties

>> Heart palpitations

>> Dizziness

>> Headache

>> Joint or muscle issues

TECHNICAL STUFF

The COVID-19 virus uses the same receptor on the human cell as the SARS virus as an entry portal into the cells of the respiratory tract. However, some amino acids in the receptor binding site are different, which may explain some differences between COVID-19 and SARS. The binding to the human target cell appears to be about 10 to 20 times stronger in COVID-19 than in the SARS agent.

Detecting a COVID-19 infection

Viruses don't give us their names or tell us they've arrived. They spread before we even know they're there — before those who contract them have symptoms and when symptoms start and are at their mildest. Testing is the way to track this invisible spread. As the virus spreads from person to person, testing helps scientists trace and contact those in the chains of transmission.

Testing has standardly been done by swabbing material from the back of the nose to look for genetic material from the virus. Testing wasn't always easy during the start of the COVID-19 pandemic. First there were no tests, and then there were not enough tests. Results took days. Lines were long.

To complicate things, some people test positive for months after the original infection. They may continue to shed pieces of the virus chewed up by their immune systems. These tiny pieces of the virus aren't infectious. The whole virus is needed to spread.

REMEMBER

More testing means better COVID-19 control. Testing lots of people avoids missing cases. Scientists look for case positivity, or the number of cases detected per number of people tested, to be quite low, hopefully even lower than 1 percent. Testing also provides guidance on when you should isolate and quarantine. Even if you're feeling well after a positive test for COVID-19, you should isolate at home for ten days. If you've been exposed to COVID-19, you should stay at home, even if you test negative, and quarantine because you may suddenly start shedding the virus, especially in the first five to seven days.

The following sections describe testing for COVID-19 and the emergence of variants.

Going through testing

Several types of tests are used to help track cases and prevent spread. They include the following:

>> **Rapid or antigen tests** look for antigens or bits of protein from the virus. Rapid tests may be less accurate than other tests. They may especially cause false negatives, where you're told you don't have it but you do. However, these false negatives are more common in those who are less infectious. They're most accurate in the first week of symptoms. Currently, rapid home tests are becoming available in pharmacies. Some use swabs in the back of the nose (nasopharyngeal), but many are a lot easier to use, relying on a swab from the front of the nose or saliva.

>> **Polymerase chain reaction (PCR) or molecular tests** test for genetic material from the virus. They're considered the "gold standard" tests and are the most accurate but take more time to give results than antigen tests. The test often look for three genes, sometimes two, that are used to make important proteins, like the spike (or S) protein. These tests usually use a nasopharyngeal swab (in the way back of the nose), but some tests use nasal, throat, or saliva samples.

>> **COVID-19 antibody tests** show whether you've previously had the virus. However, having COVID-19 once doesn't protect you from all future exposures and variants, so it's important to realize testing positive doesn't mean you're immune forever from COVID-19 or from new variants. These tests use blood samples.

Recognizing variants

Testing also includes sampling to track for new variants. Each variant is just a different branch in the COVID-19 family tree. Every time a virus makes copies of itself, it can change slightly. Over time, small changes collect and together cause bigger changes, making these branches more distinct. These bigger changes mean some variants can behave differently than the COVID-19 we are used to. They may spread more easily between people or cause more deaths. They may make it more likely that you will catch COVID-19 a second time. They may also cause different symptoms, and some may even be harder to find on some tests. Variants initially occur locally, but if they spread more easily, they may replace existing variants and spread elsewhere.

REMEMBER

Variants can also make certain vaccines less effective, although the 2021 vaccines seem a good match against the current variants. Many variants survive only a short time before fading out, while others become the dominant type in one area but not in others. Continued testing will help researchers stay up to date on new COVID-19 variants and their possible complications.

New variants can differ from old school SARS-CoV-2 in a few different ways. Usually they cause only one or two different changes. These might include

>> Spreading more easily person to person

>> Causing more re-infections in those who have already had COVID-19

>> Causing more severe illness and more deaths

>> Leading to more breakthrough infections after certain vaccines

>> Changing symptoms experienced (less loss of smell, more sore throats)

>> Making it harder to identify the virus with certain tests (if the gene or protein tested for is very different from what the test looks for)

There are Variants of Concern, which the World Health Organization and the U.S. Centers for Disease Control and Prevention (CDC) consider the most important ones to watch. These have had the biggest changes from the original SARS-CoV-2 we saw, and these are changes we are concerned about:

>> Alpha was the first concerning new variant identified. It was first called B.1.1.7 and was seen to be more transmissible and cause more severe illness. It first spread in Great Britain and then spread to Ireland, Portugal, and elsewhere, causing sudden steep surges. It has spread to the United States, where it displaced other variants, but fortunately by then, vaccination rates were higher and helped protect against this variant.

>> Beta was identified just after Alpha. It was called B.1.351 when it was first seen in South Africa. It wasn't that it caused more transmission. It's that it caused folks who had COVID-19 before to get sick again. Those who had previously had COVID-19 (and had antibodies) were just as likely to get this new variant as anyone else. This variant then spread to other countries in Africa.

>> Gamma was first seen in Brazil. It showed itself to be a mix of both transmissibility and immune evasion. It was more transmissible (though not as much as Alpha) and able to evade immunity (though not as much as Beta). It struck a city in the Amazon (Manaus) that had already been through a horrible epidemic. It was thought three in four had been infected before this variant showed up. Once this variant appeared, the surge was even greater than before, with even more deaths. This variant traveled to Peru, where it caused another huge surge where already three in four had been infected. It continued to spread in other parts of South America, causing more surges. It spread to Uruguay, which up until then had been able to keep COVID-19 largely at bay through public health measures. It then spread to Chile, which had one of the highest rates of vaccination at the time but still faced a surge, as vaccination had not yet reached herd immunity levels.

>> Delta was found to be a variant that both was more transmissible than all other variants (including Alpha) and can escape immunity (though less than Beta). This variant has spread through India and nearby countries, causing huge surges and many deaths. As this variant is more transmissible, it replaced Alpha where Alpha first dominated in Great Britain. It was also seen to cause some breakthrough infections with vaccines, but more so with those who had only one of two doses.

REMEMBER

We will continue to learn more about these variants. Each day there is more news. What we thought we knew today about variants may not be what we know tomorrow.

There are many other variants out there. There have been new variants that have developed in California and New York and were associated with continued spread in the United States.

REMEMBER

More mutations will pop up and more variants will appear if SARS-CoV-2 continues to spread. As long as many are not vaccinated around the world, SARS-CoV-2 will continue to spread.

Digging into the development of COVID-19 vaccines

There are vaccines for COVID-19. This alone is cause for celebration. This is pretty amazing.

It took a lot of science to get us here, but vaccines will make all the difference in countries' opening up and getting back to normal living. Many different types of vaccines have already been developed. Around the world, over 100 vaccines have been in COVID-19 vaccine trials. Vaccines may be approved and used in some countries and not others.

REMEMBER

Even though the development process was rapid, these vaccines went through all the same trials other vaccines have. They went through Phase I and then II and then III. (We talk about the vaccine clinical trials and how they work in Chapter 5.) COVID-19 vaccines are probably the most watched vaccines to ever be studied. So many different researchers, governments, and groups have poured through all the data to come out.

Less than one year after this virus started to spread, we had a vaccine. In the first six months of vaccine rollout in the United States, three vaccines were in use in the United States. All three are highly effective. They showed high efficacy in trials, demonstrating again and again that they prevented almost all deaths and the large majority of cases. These vaccines have continued to perform effectively, even as new variants arrive.

Most of these vaccines use the spike protein on the outside of the coronavirus that gave it its name — the crowned virus. What was so memorable to Dr. June Almeida is also memorable to our immune system.

The first vaccine to be rolled out in the United States was an mRNA (messenger ribonucleic acid). It was the first time an mRNA vaccine was used. The vaccine gives our bodies the instructions on how to make that recognizable spike protein. It's a bit like buying furniture that has to be assembled. The vaccine has bits of mRNA, which are instructions telling our cells how to make the spike protein. Then our immune system will recognize the virus if it's ever exposed because it will see those spikes that are still so recognizable, whether to our immune system or Dr. June Almeida.

These mRNA vaccines are also the Snapchat of vaccines. The mRNA does not last long; it's fragile. It needs to be protected in a fatty coat to get it to its destination. This means if we track this vaccine, it only goes as far as the closest lymph nodes to where you had the injection. It doesn't travel any further. It doesn't spread throughout our bodies and definitely doesn't go near a fetus in someone who is pregnant.

The first mRNA vaccine that was given emergency authorization in the United States was the Pfizer vaccine. This was quickly followed by the Moderna vaccine, which is quite similar. Both of these vaccines require two doses, spaced either three or four weeks apart.

There's also now a vaccine that requires just one dose — the Johnson & Johnson vaccine. This vaccine uses a viral vector. The virus, here an adenovirus, can bring the same instructions on how to make a spike protein. Instead of these instructions for assembly coming from mRNA safely tucked away in a fatty cushion, these instructions are carried in a virus. This virus doesn't make a copy of itself and doesn't spread. Instead, the virus just delivers the instructions, and our bodies have a new copy of the spike protein with a warning that this protein is trouble, and we'd better watch out if we ever see it.

All three of these vaccines make a spike protein that's a bit different than it is in the typical virus. Proteins are made up of chains of amino acids, their basic building block. Proteins, though, don't look like necklaces. They twist and bend as different amino acids create different bends and attract and repel each other. In this case, the spike protein in the vaccine has two added amino acids called *prolines*. These amino acids create a stiff bend in the protein, letting it take a slightly different shape. The shape it takes is the shape it naturally takes when it's about to enter the cell. This lets our immune system best recognize this virus when it's about to attack us.

Other vaccines are being used around the world. There are inactivated, whole killed vaccines that include the whole virus. There are vaccines that just use that spike protein alone, no assembly required. There are other viral vector vaccines, including the Oxford/AstraZeneca vaccine, which have been distributed in the United Kingdom and Europe and also in Africa, Asia, and South America.

The COVID-19 vaccines have made a huge difference so far. These vaccines will make an even bigger difference if even more people are vaccinated in every city, every state, every country, and every continent.

Before vaccination, about half of those hospitalized and 85 percent of those who died were elderly. Once vaccinations picked up, the elderly were the first vaccinated, and suddenly the elderly were better off. Their infections and deaths were at much lower rates than their younger neighbors. Vaccines make a difference.

It will be important for large numbers of people to be vaccinated to have the vaccines not only protect us as individuals, but also protect our communities and countries at large. This requires ensuring that everyone has access to the vaccines, understands the risks and benefits, and feels comfortable taking these vaccines, without hesitancy. Many around the world have not been able to easily access these vaccines. If we're able to ensure the world is well vaccinated, we can eventually move past having COVID-19 loom over us.

Dealing with vaccine side effects

Side effects can occur with any vaccine. The COVID-19 vaccines, particularly the mRNA vaccines, are considered *reactogenic,* which means that physical symptoms can occur after the vaccine. When you take a tetanus or shingles vaccine, you may feel a bit under the weather for a day or so. Same here.

After you have the COVID-19 vaccine, especially an mRNA vaccine, you may not be able to move your arm for a day or two. You may feel tired or have a headache. You may have to take a day or two off school or work. But that's usually it. (We review the known side effects and current ingredients in the COVID-19 vaccines in detail in Chapter 10.)

Some people have allergic reactions to the vaccines. The mRNA vaccines come coated in a fatty little carrying case. Without this protective layer, the mRNA would just fall apart and disappear. This layer is made up of something we often have in our bathrooms — polyethylene glycol. It's what makes up MiraLAX — an anti-constipation medication. It's also in our toothpaste and shampoo.

TIP

Some of us — and very few of us — can have an allergy to polyethylene glycol or something else in the vaccine, which can even cause anaphylaxis (with shortness of breath, throat swelling, and low blood pressure). This can certainly be a worry, but it doesn't happen often; it occurs in about two to five of 1 million people and usually happens in the first 15 to 30 minutes after the vaccination, so most people wait 15 minutes after getting it to be sure, and those who know they have allergies can wait a little longer.

Blood clots have been reported with two of the viral vector vaccines — Johnson & Johnson and the Oxford/AstraZeneca vaccine. There were cases of both clotting and bleeding. The bleeding was due to having low levels of platelets, the cell fragments that help blood clot. This, though, was rare — for Johnson & Johnson, it occurred in about one case in 1 million overall. There's a two-in-a-million chance of being struck by lightning. The risk for blood clots was higher among young women, though, especially those under 50 years old. This risk may be closer to seven in 1 million or even a bit higher for some younger women. It also occurred more frequently with the Oxford/AstraZeneca vaccine, in about one in 75,000 people, though much more commonly, again, in young women.

There was a pause on these vaccines in the spring of 2021 while the problem was studied. It was decided the risk of COVID-19 outweighed a risk that wasn't much more, on average, than being hit by lightning, but the study did highlight the issue for especially young women who are at higher risk. Some countries have recommended these vaccines be used only in older adults.

There have been lots of rumors about side effects from these vaccines. Many have been afraid that side effects can affect fertility or pregnancy. In fact, the first trials of these vaccines asked participants not to get pregnant, but of course some did. The same number became pregnant in each arm of the trial. Those who received the vaccine were just as likely to get pregnant as those who did not. Moreover, studies on male fertility and in IVF (in vitro fertilization) clinics showed no change. There was, however, an impact on fertility, especially among men, from getting COVID-19 itself.

REMEMBER

Now that millions of people have had the vaccines, there will be people who have bad outcomes after being vaccinated. Vaccines don't give us a pass from all bad things in life. COVID-19 vaccines just protect us against COVID-19. It's always important to make sure any potential side effect is actually more common than it would have been otherwise. If you study enough people, a few will have some unexpected problems. The original Moderna vaccine trial had one participant who was hit by lightning. And we certainly don't think that this vaccine increases the risk of being struck by lightning.

Aiming for herd immunity

REMEMBER

What's so great about vaccines is that they don't just keep you from getting sick, they help you keep everyone from getting sick. The more people who are vaccinated, the less likely a virus can spread from person to person. This is *herd immunity,* which is obtained when a certain percentage of a population is vaccinated, depending on how transmissible the virus is. It becomes like a force shield that the virus can't penetrate. But if only a small number of people are vaccinated, it just won't do much to stop the virus from jumping from one person to another.

There's not one herd immunity goal. It is a bit of a moving target. The estimate of the percent needed to be vaccinated for herd immunity is $1 - 1/R0$. *Ro* is the number of cases one case would lead to if everyone was susceptible. For measles, which has an R0 between 12 and 18, herd immunity requires about 95 percent to be vaccinated. Thing is, R0 is just an estimation. It is not a fixed number. There are different factors that go into it.

TECHNICAL STUFF

Roughly, the following applies:

R0 = Beta * c * d

R0 = (Beta — rate of transmission per contact) * (c — number of contacts per time) * (d — duration of time remains infectious)

This means as these factors change, R0 changes:

>> Transmissibility can change with new variants or reduced mask use.

>> Contacts can change when people begin mixing more.

>> Duration of infectiousness can change when people don't stay home when they are exposed (quarantine) or sick (isolation).

The number who need to be vaccinated is very different based on what the world is like. Fewer need to be vaccinated if we are having a limited number of contacts and schools are closed, but if we want to get back to life where there are concerts and all universities are fully open, we need more people vaccinated. Vaccines also aren't perfect; there can be breakthrough infections. As such, the efficacy of the vaccine should also be accounted for. There's also the chance that, no matter how effective the vaccine is, some people do not respond to the vaccine as well and immunity may wear off, so we need a bit of a buffer. Estimates are that between 70 percent and 90 percent will need to be vaccinated to start activating that force shield. Cases, though, will become less common as more people become vaccinated, even if we haven't reached these thresholds to provide protection to everyone.

Getting vaccinated is not just about yourself. It's about helping your community. Some folks won't respond to a vaccine as easily as others. Those who have a weaker immune system — because they have had an organ transplant or are on cancer treatment or on dialysis for their kidneys — just may not make as strong a response to the vaccine. That's why we need herd immunity, so that everyone is protected by vaccines even if the vaccine won't protect them as well.

There are also delays around the world in ensuring everyone is vaccinated. There just aren't enough vaccines, and they aren't getting everywhere they are needed. As COVID-19 continues to spread, unchecked by vaccines, the virus can take more lives and create new variants, creating even more problems for a longer period of time.

There's another problem vaccines face: their own success. The more successful a vaccine is, the less people may feel they need it. We make many vaccines routine and required for schools because if lots of people just didn't get around to getting vaccinated, we'd have to start thinking about measles and polio and all sorts of diseases again. Vaccination helps us put COVID-19 behind us.

Having had COVID-19 before still means you should get vaccinated now. Natural immunity is not as robust against new variants. Herd immunity has not been achieved by natural infections. New variants can spread where communities have already been hit hard by COVID-19. In South Africa, it was found that the Beta variant (B.1.351) was just as likely to infect you, whether or not you had antibodies to the first type of COVID-19 that had spread. In parts of Brazil and Peru, over three in four were thought to have been infected, and there was then a surge, described as bigger than the first. Having had COVID-19 before was not enough to stop this new variant, known as the Gamma variant (P.1) spread. Other countries have also seen the devastating consequences of allowing COVID-19 to spread without intervention. Although many get better from COVID-19, the consequences are severe for some from COVID-19 — whether death or long COVID.

Keeping safe from COVID-19 if you're not yet protected by vaccination

It's important to remember to keep safe from COVID-19 if you are not yet vaccinated or your immune system does not respond to the vaccine. This is a virus that spreads mostly through the air, as droplets and aerosols and much less through contact with contaminated objects.

To keep safe from COVID-19, do the following:

>> Get vaccinated, if you haven't. This is the single most effective way to prevent COVID-19.

>> Practice *social distancing*. That means staying at least 6 feet (2 meters) away from others and not hugging or shaking hands.

>> Most transmission occurs indoors. Take advantage of any nice weather and see friends, visit family, and even have meetings outdoors.

>> Open multiple windows and doors (if it's safe to do so) to let fresh air in.

>> If you have portable fans, point them away from people. Set them near the window to blow air out. Exhaust fans in the bathroom and above the stove can also help if you have visitors.

>> If you have ceiling fans, set them to draw air upwards.

>> If you do have a central HVAC (heating, ventilation, and air conditioning) system, you can use this to improve indoor ventilation. Be sure it is set to draw air from outdoors and is not set to recirculate.

>> Avoid crowds (including private meetings).

>> If you haven't been vaccinated, wear a face mask. A homemade cloth mask is generally fine for protecting others. Check out www.cdc.gov/coronavirus/2019-ncov/prevent-getting-sick/diy-cloth-face-coverings.html for details.

>> Avoid touching your face.

>> Do not sneeze in your hand; use the crook of your elbow instead.

>> Wash your hands. Be aware that frequently touched surfaces — like door-knobs and countertops — can be the source of viruses, though maybe just cold viruses.

TIP

Comprehensive recommendations for conduct can be found at the Center for Disease Control website, www.cdc.gov/coronavirus/2019-ncov/index.html.

Coping with COVID-19 and flu season

As fully vaccinated people take off their masks and start to mingle, all those cold viruses start mingling too. A whole lot of kids didn't get their preschool colds due to social distancing. With more kids whose immune systems have never seen the standard colds before, a lot more colds will be going around.

The same holds true for the flu. As the world emerges from COVID-19, it's a good time to get the flu vaccine. The flu is no fun. It feels awful, and it likely takes between one-quarter and half a million lives each year as it circles the globe. It will also be a lot harder for doctors and nurses to figure out who has the flu, who has COVID-19, and who has a cold as outbreaks occur and all these different viruses spread.

REMEMBER

We have vaccines for the flu and now COVID-19. Both save many lives as well as prevent seasonal misery. Now we just need to finish the work of the Common Cold Unit and find ways to stop cold viruses from spreading as well.

Chapter **4**

Bacterial Bad Guys

B acteria are all around us. They're in the air, the soil, and the water. They're inside of us, too. They're in our guts, on our skin, and in our mouths. We have more cells inside of us that are bacterial than human. Many of these bacteria aren't a problem at all, and many we'd be worse off without.

Bacterial infections used to be a much greater problem. Clean water and better living conditions have helped prevent some bacterial infections. But even more importantly, vaccines and antibiotics have changed the way we fight bacteria. Thanks to antibiotics, some infections that were once deadly are now easily treatable. But more importantly, vaccines prevent some infections from ever happening.

This chapter discusses what makes bacteria different from viruses. We explain how vaccines prevent bacterial infections and help us save antibiotics. We also dive into how vaccines work against certain bacteria.

Understanding What Makes Bacteria Different from Viruses

Bacteria and viruses both make us sick, sometimes with many of the same symptoms. Some viruses, like norovirus and rotavirus, cause diarrhea; so do some bacteria, like cholera and typhoid. Some bacteria, like pertussis and pneumococcus, can cause coughs, as do some viruses like influenza and COVID-19.

We can't always tell without more testing whether an infection is bacterial or viral. But sometimes we can. Most colds are due to viruses. Cellulitis, an infection of the skin, is almost always due to bacteria.

What makes bacteria fundamentally different from viruses is that bacteria are alive and viruses are not:

>> Viruses aren't alive. They don't have cells. They just have genetic material (their assembly instructions) tucked away inside a shell. Viruses can make copies of themselves only if they hijack a cell and control the cell's own machinery to make copies.

>> Bacteria are a lot more complex. They have cells. These cells are full of the machinery they need to make all that they need and break down food for energy.

Almost all bacteria can make copies of themselves outside of our cells. They have all they need to make new copies of themselves. There are a few exceptions, like chlamydia, which have to be inside other cells to reproduce. Some other bacteria can reproduce outside of our cells but may enter our cells to cause disease (like the bacteria that cause gonorrhea and tuberculosis, or TB), and many others cause disease from outside or a mix of both, like staph aureus and E. coli.

Digging into Vaccines That Defuse Bacteria

Vaccines provide that "Wanted" photo of what our immune system needs to hunt down the bacteria if it ever arrives. A vaccine may include a whole bacteria that has been killed. This type is less common now, but the injectable typhoid vaccine and some oral cholera vaccines are made this way.

In the past, whole-cell vaccines were used for pertussis, but now an acellular vaccine is used. (An *acellular vaccine* contains cellular material but not complete cells.) A vaccine can also include a whole and live, but attenuated or mild, bacteria that is related to the target bacteria but not quite the same, such as those used for TB (BCG), cholera (oral Vaxchora vaccine), and typhoid (oral Vivotif). The vaccine can also include just bits of the outside of the bacteria. A conjugate vaccine can include a piece of a weak antigen from the bacteria tied to a strong reminder, a strong antigen.

Polysaccharide vaccines are made of long chains of sugars that can be found on the outside of some bacteria and are used to prevent pneumococcus (which can cause pneumonia, meningitis, or a bloodstream infection), meningococcus (which can cause meningitis or a bloodstream infection), and Salmonella Typhi (which can cause typhoid with diarrhea and bloodstream infections).

The following sections cover how vaccines work against bacteria and the bacterial diseases that you can fight off with vaccines.

The make-up of vaccines that protect against bacterial toxins

Some vaccines are based on the very toxins that cause us harm. These vaccines use a harmless but similar version of the toxin (or poison) that some bacteria release — this toxin is what causes disease. The harmless version of the toxin is called a *toxoid.* The toxoid then becomes the antigen or "Wanted" photo for our immune system. Based on this protein toxoid, our immune system knows how to prepare an immune response to the toxin.

These vaccines do not create as strong and long lasting a response as some vaccines. The toxoid usually needs to be paired with an adjuvant, like aluminum or calcium salts. These vaccines usually require several doses, and we may need boosters throughout our lives. (See Chapter 5 for more on adjuvants and other vaccine ingredients.)

These vaccines are both safe and stable. The toxoids cannot *replicate,* or make copies of themselves, or spread. The toxoids also can't change or somehow become the poisonous toxin. The toxoid vaccines are usually very stable and can be stored in different conditions, including being exposed to various temperatures, humidity levels, and amounts of sunlight.

The bacterial illnesses that vaccines prevent

What's so important about vaccines is that they prevent infections from ever happening. This means no one needs to get sick or suffer if a vaccine has been created to prevent their infection. Vaccines are approved in the United States to prevent ten different bacterial illnesses: anthrax, cholera, diphtheria, haemophilus influenzae type b, meningococcus, pertussis, pneumococcus, tetanus, tuberculosis, and typhoid.

Anthrax

Anthrax is a rod-shaped bacteria known as *Bacillus anthracis.* The disease and its prevention gained attention in the United States after anthrax was sent through the mail in 2001 as a bioterrorism plot. In reality, it's really the poorest farmers, far from the United States, who come into the most contact with the bacteria. It's found in soil and can be contracted by people who ingest the anthrax spores in food, in water, or from the air, or through a break in the skin. It can cause contact anthrax (skin infection), injection anthrax (with contaminated injections), gastrointestinal anthrax, and inhalation anthrax (the most serious, caused by breathing in the spores in the air).

Anthrax is often associated with infected livestock outside of the United States where the infection persists. It can be due to direct contact with an infected animal (contact anthrax) or ingestion of contaminated meat (gastrointestinal anthrax). Spores also can fly into the air and be swallowed after playing drums from a contaminated animal hide.

For most people, anthrax isn't a concern, and the vaccine isn't routinely given, except to certain military personnel, people who work in laboratories with the bacteria, or those who work with animals potentially infected with it. Anthrax isn't contagious from person to person.

Cholera

The cholera vaccine isn't given routinely in the United States. It is given for travel. Cholera persists year after year in the waters in some countries and has surged, somewhat unexpectedly, in other countries where sanitation resources were insufficient to keep drinking water protected from stool contamination when the bacteria was introduced.

The disease is caused by the bacterium *Vibrio cholerae* serogroup O1 or O139. It causes profuse diarrhea that looks like rice water. It is caused by swallowing the bacteria and an infection develops with the intestines (but not the rest of the body). There are no fevers. The symptoms appear suddenly, usually two to three days after exposure.

Those who have more acid in their stomachs will have a bit of protection. Most will recover with oral rehydration with clean water containing salt and sugar. Cholera usually lasts only a few days. Around 10 percent of people infected become severely ill. Some will need intravenous fluids. In rare cases — usually less than 1 percent if rehydration is easily available — severe diarrhea, vomiting, and dehydration can lead to death from cholera in hours.

Cholera still infects nearly 3 million people each year worldwide and kills almost 100,000. The bacteria is spread through fecal material in water or in infected food. If you're traveling to places with poor sanitation and hygiene, your medical provider may recommend you get vaccinated against cholera.

Diphtheria

Diphtheria used to be known as the "strangling angel" of children. It causes a terrible and painful neck swelling with a film inside the throat called a *pseudomembrane.* Unable to breathe, children gasp for breath and die. The disease is so awful that it's the reason intubation was invented. It's really a terrible disease to ever see, and it still affects thousands of children today in some parts of the world.

The disease is caused by a toxin released by the bacteria called *Corynebacterium diphtheriae.* The most notable effects are the swelling in the neck, swollen lymph nodes, and the pseudomembrane that make it difficult to breathe. The toxin can also damage the heart, kidneys, and nervous system. Those who are infected are often children but can also be adults.

For those with serious infections, intubation is often needed. Antibiotics can help treat the infection but sometimes not quickly enough when breathing is difficult. Antitoxin, or antibodies, can also be given to reduce, but not eliminate, the risk of death.

WARNING

Infections are almost always transmitted from other people, by way of droplets in the air or by direct contact. The bacteria can live in the nose or throat of healthy people. Some people who have immunity to the bacteria, whether through vaccination or an infection, may carry the disease anyway. They may carry the bacteria that can infect others but have no symptoms. So it's really important to have everyone vaccinated while this bacteria is still out there; otherwise, an unsuspecting parent may pass the infection on to their child.

Although based on the toxin, the vaccine itself isn't dangerous. A series of six vaccinations is given during infancy and childhood. (Chapter 8 has details on vaccines for children.) The vaccines have been very successful in eliminating diphtheria infections where resources are plentiful. Local infections of diphtheria have been eliminated in the United States.

In some parts of the world, where the needed series of vaccinations is not available or completed, outbreaks of this terrible infection still occur. As long as diphtheria remains a problem anywhere in the world, it can travel and infect those who are not vaccinated. The last case caught in the United States was in an adult who had not travelled for many years but whose spouse had recently traveled back from an area with a diphtheria outbreak and had no symptoms. Chapter 6 has more on diphtheria.

Haemophilus influenzae type b (Hib)

Although it sounds like a virus because of the influenzae part of its name, this mouthful of a name is actually a bacteria, often shortened to Hib. Hib causes many types of infections, often in children, but sometimes in susceptible adults as well. Hib can cause diseases as diverse as ear infections; infections of the heart, bones, and joints; and pneumonia.

Before the development of the vaccine, Hib was the leading cause of bacterial meningitis in children age 5, affecting around 20,000 children each year. Because of this, Hib vaccinations are given in a series started early, at age 2 months. The vaccine, first developed in the late 1980s, has virtually eliminated Hib infections in children. (Flip to Chapter 6 for details on Hib.)

Meningococcus

The meningococcus vaccine prevents bacteria called *Neisseria meningitidis*, also known as meningococcus, from causing illnesses such as meningitis or blood infections. Meningococcal diseases mainly affect infants, children, and teens. College campuses, military barracks, and other areas packed with teens and young adults are notoriously risky for meningococcal outbreaks.

Meningococcal infections cause meningitis, characterized by fever, stiff neck, severe headache, light sensitivity, and vomiting. The infections often cause long-term damage, as well as killing between 10 and 15 percent of people who become infected. See Chapter 6 for more information.

Pertussis

Pertussis, better known as whooping cough, can last from two to eight weeks. Caused by the bacterium *Bordetella*, whooping cough is extremely contagious and normally affects children. Babies who are infected in their first six months may have an infection deep in their lungs. They may not cough but may have periods during which they stop breathing. One in two babies infected needs to be hospitalized. Whooping cough hasn't disappeared in the United States; the largest outbreak recently affected over 48,000 people. Flip to Chapter 6 for details on pertussis.

Pneumococcus

The *Streptococcus pneumoniae* bacteria can cause a number of different infections, including infections of the lungs, blood, ears, and meninges. These bacterial infections are most dangerous in the very young and very old, and can be fatal. Around one in 20 persons with pneumococcal pneumonia dies from it; pneumococcal meningitis kills one in 12 children infected and one in seven older adults infected. Head to Chapter 6 for more info.

Tetanus

Tetanus is known as lockjaw. The toxin from tetanus can cause muscles to contract painfully. These muscles spasm and lock up. This can happen in the jaw, making it hard to open the mouth or swallow. This can also make it hard to breathe. Breathing becomes shallow. It's hard to see that someone is struggling to breathe as they begin to breathe slower and slower, unable to speak or shout for help. Those suffering from this painful disease often have contracted facial muscles that make it look as if they're grinning or smiling. This can also make it hard to breathe. It's an awful disease to see. It can be caused by a simple child's injury or a fall off a motorcycle or an injury on a building site.

Treatment can require prolonged intubation, along with an antibiotic and antitoxin. There isn't a simple cure.

The disease can't spread from person to person. It's caused by a bacteria, *Clostridium tetani,* which produces spores. These bacteria are found in the environment, usually in soil. Rusty nails are often blamed, but it's actually the dirt and dust that get in the nail, rather than the nail or rust, that harbor the bacteria. The bacteria can get into a dirty wound, a puncture from a needle or a nail, a burn, when someone is partly crushed by something heavy, or even a nonsterile injection.

WARNING

Those who haven't finished their childhood vaccinations or who haven't had a recent vaccine are most likely to be at risk. A wound contaminated by dirt is also more likely to lead to tetanus in those who aren't fully vaccinated. Those who have diabetes are at greater risk, as are those who are on immune-suppressing medications or who use injection drugs. Only very rarely does tetanus develop in someone who is vaccinated.

The tetanus vaccine is a toxoid vaccine and is combined with the diphtheria vaccine. It's often combined with a pertussis vaccine as well. Check out Chapter 6 for details.

Tuberculosis

Mycobacterium tuberculosis, the bacteria that causes tuberculosis (TB), travels through the air. Tuberculosis affects mainly the lungs, but it can also affect the spine, brain, intestines, kidneys, or just about any other part of the body. Fever, cough, and unexplained weight loss and night sweats are the most common symptoms. In the 1600s to 1800s in Europe, as well as in the United States, TB accounted for one in four deaths. Using public health measures — improved living conditions, better ventilation, isolation — TB cases dropped in the United States, even further with treatment.

Cases of tuberculosis have dropped consistently in the United States over the past decades; around 71 percent of cases occur in people born outside the United States. However, worldwide, TB is the world's greatest infectious disease killer. Year after year, more people die from TB than anything else. Today, the vaccine is only given to people in the United States with certain risk factors.

Typhoid

Around 27 million people worldwide are infected each year by the Salmonella Typhi bacteria, including around 350 in the United States, most of whom have traveled out of the country to areas where typhoid is still endemic, like parts of Africa, India, and Southeast Asia. This bacteria is usually passed through the fecal-oral route. It causes fevers and abdominal pain, and can cause diarrhea and constipation. It can be treated by antibiotics but is often not diagnosed correctly, and now the bacteria is growing resistant to most antibiotics used. The typhoid vaccines (oral and injectable) are only 50 to 80 percent effective against the disease and need to be repeated frequently (every three years).

Comparing Antibiotics and Vaccines

When you're sick, you just want to take something to make you better. So some people will take antibiotics for viral infections. The thing is, antibiotics don't make viral infections better. Usually, you get better anyway because many common viral infections make you sick for only a few days whether you take anything or not. But then you think it's the antibiotics that did the trick. And the next time you have a viral infection, you want to take antibiotics again.

In some cases, taking antibiotics can be appropriate if you have a viral infection. Some viral infections are more likely to be followed by bacterial disease. For example, sometimes the damage that the flu does to your lungs can put you at risk for developing a bacterial superinfection. Measles infection can weaken your immune system and put you at risk for a bacterial infection. People vaccinated against measles are found to be less likely to have a serious bacterial infection.

REMEMBER

You may wonder, "If antibiotics treat bacteria, why do we need vaccines?" The answer is simple. Vaccines *prevent* bacterial infections. Antibiotics only *treat* the disease once you have it. That's like choosing between a superpower to prevent all dangerous fires and asking firefighters to put out out-of-control fires. You still get sick, and the antibiotics don't always work. Antibiotics are used only when you're ill, and sometimes doctors don't know which antibiotics will work, or the antibiotics that used to work no longer do. Not every bacterial infection will melt away with antibiotics. Vaccines are a bit of a superpower and let us deflect bacteria before they ever make us sick.

WARNING

The more we use antibiotics, the more we lose them. What used to be treated by penicillin now isn't always able to be. We can't just take antibiotics again and again and expect them to keep working. Antibiotics select out the bacteria that can resist them. It's a bit like using weedkiller. The first few times it works, but then the weeds that grow are just those that can resist the weedkiller.

WARNING

Antibiotics also can have all sorts of side effects that we don't have with vaccines. Antibiotics can cause diarrhea by wiping out the normal bacteria of our guts. This can lead to the overgrowth of a bacteria we really don't like called C Diff (*Clostridium difficile*), which can cause a very bad case of diarrhea and for some can cause hospitalization, a need for surgery, and even death. Other antibiotics can sometimes make our heart beat funny, causing arrhythmias or even sudden death. Some can cause severe sunburns. Others can damage our tendons. Still others can cause liver problems or severe allergies and skin reactions.

About 100 to 500 in 1 million people who take penicillin have a severe allergic reaction called *anaphylaxis,* which can cause them to stop breathing. Although some vaccines can cause allergies and anaphylaxis, the number of people affected is a lot fewer. Anaphylaxis is about 1.3 in 1 million on average with vaccines.

Seeing How Vaccines Help Prevent Antibiotic Resistance

We are quickly losing antibiotics, as we note in the previous section. What used to be easily treated by penicillin or another antibiotic may not be treatable by any antibiotics or only by a few specific ones. This can require waiting for tests that take days to tell us which antibiotics work, which can be very dangerous when someone has a serious bacterial infection. What used to require a simple pill now requires infusions in the hospital. We often speak of medicine before antibiotics, before penicillin was discovered in 1928. Some scientists speak of a coming time that is post-antibiotics.

Currently, in the United States, 2.8 million people develop an antibiotic-resistant infection and 35,000 die from one each year. Worldwide, the 700,000 deaths a year to antibiotic-resistant bacterial infections is expected to rise to 10 million a year by 2050. Antibiotic resistance is growing, and it's a worrisome problem.

Vaccines, both bacterial and viral, help prevent antibiotic resistance. How's that?

>> Bacterial vaccines can prevent the need for antibiotics in the first place. Vaccination for pneumococcus has led to a reduction in antibiotic serotypes that were resistant to antibiotics but couldn't resist vaccination. We also often use the wrong antibiotic for bacterial infections, and this extra exposure to antibiotics can create resistant strains without any benefit.

>> Viral vaccines can prevent symptoms that are often mistaken for bacteria. People often take antibiotics for viruses. Colds are usually caused by viruses, but many people take antibiotics for them even though they don't help. The bacteria in our guts, skin, and elsewhere are then exposed to antibiotics, and the bacteria that can resist the antibiotics are more likely to survive and thrive, leading to us having more resistant bacteria. Bacteria can also mix and match genes and can spread resistant genes to other bacteria.

2

Verifying Valuable Vaccines

IN THIS PART . . .

Discover the three types of vaccines and study the vaccine approval process.

Find a list of the current vaccines available.

Understand what to expect when you get a vaccine and become aware of side effects.

Chapter **5**

Distinguishing and Testing Different Vaccines

Although people sometimes talk about vaccines as if they were all the same, vaccines created to prevent different diseases are — well, different.

You can think of vaccines as a kind of "Wanted" picture for your immune system. Vaccines give your immune system a snapshot of the *pathogen* — the scientific name for the bacteria, virus, parasite, or fungi that make us ill — to remember it by. Not all "Wanted" pictures are the same. Some vaccines may show the entire pathogen to the immune system. Some may show a pathogen that looks almost the same. Others may give a picture of a key identifying feature, like a tattoo.

In this chapter, we explain how vaccines are alike — and how they're different. We explain why certain vaccines are used for some illnesses and why we use other types for different ones. Often, the reason for different types of vaccines comes down to the development of new and better technology. We also describe the processes used to create vaccines.

We also take you into the world of clinical trials: the complicated process of setting them up and carrying them out, and the importance of making sure you — and millions of others — have the most effective and safest vaccine possible.

Getting to Know the Different Types of Vaccines

Vaccines fall into two broad categories: whole-pathogen vaccines and subunit vaccines. They're further subdivided into several other categories, including live vaccines, inactivated vaccines, toxoid vaccines, nucleic acid vaccines, and viral vector vaccines. This may seem unnecessarily complicated — can't science come up with just one type of vaccine that covers a multitude of diseases? The answer is, no they can't, in most cases, although there are some vaccines that can be combined into one injection.

In this section, we look at the types of vaccines available today and the reason why certain vaccines are made the way they are. Most importantly, we explain how specific vaccines may affect you.

Whole-pathogen vaccines

REMEMBER

A *whole-pathogen vaccine* is made from — no surprise here — the whole germ that makes you ill. To continue the "Wanted" poster analogy we start earlier in this chapter, whole-pathogen vaccines are like a "Wanted" poster that shows the whole person. In the same way, whole-pathogen vaccines show your immune system a weakened (live) or dead (inactivated) version of the pathogen. In some cases, a vaccine provides a picture of a very similar pathogen, the way a "Wanted" poster may show a sketch rather than an actual person.

TECHNICAL STUFF

Scientists aren't resting on their laurels when it comes to creating vaccines. Vaccines of the future may be able to attack cancer cells before they spread, or to prevent complications from diseases such as HIV from occurring.

Looking at live vaccines

Live vaccines are made from weakened or similar versions of the germs that cause disease. These bacterial or viral strains are weakened in the laboratory and cause usually no, or else few, symptoms when they're given to you.

After just one or two doses, these vaccines may protect you for years or even a lifetime. They create a long-lasting immune response much like a natural infection would, just minus the worrisome disease. These are some of science's oldest vaccines. They are tried-and-true, and in some cases, having been used for many decades.

WARNING

There are a few downsides to live vaccines, however. Because they contain a weakened but live germ — also called an *attenuated virus or bacteria* — they may give you mild symptoms. Some people shouldn't take these vaccines. Some immune systems aren't ready to handle these attenuated vaccines, but some immune systems, even if maybe a bit weakened, can.

You should talk to your doctor about whether these vaccines are right for you if you

>> Have a compromised immune system

>> Are being treated for cancer

>> Are taking immune suppressive drugs for an autoimmune disorder

>> Have had an organ transplant

>> Have advanced HIV

If you might be pregnant, talk to your doctor. In general, live vaccines are not recommended in pregnancy. The exception is the yellow fever vaccine, if you live in or are traveling to an area where this illness is prevalent.

WARNING

Live vaccines have two other potential drawbacks:

>> They have to be kept cool before they're administered, so they may not be practical where adequate refrigeration is limited.

>> Sometimes immunity doesn't last as long as expected and you may not know you need to be re-vaccinated.

Live vaccines include chicken pox, measles, mumps, rubella (sometimes called German measles), oral polio, and, in the past, smallpox vaccines. Tuberculosis, oral typhoid, and oral cholera vaccines are live bacteria vaccines. The yellow fever vaccine is also a live vaccine.

Some of these — measles, mumps, and rubella, called the MMR vaccine, or MMR along with chicken pox (varicella), called the MMRV— can be combined and given in one injection (but you need at least two doses). The MMRV is more commonly given now. We cover the development of specific vaccines later in this chapter.

REMEMBER

Most new vaccines are not live vaccines. The current live vaccines have a good safety profile, but they are tried-and-true. Scientists also want a vaccine that works for everyone, including pregnant women and people with compromised immune systems. There's also the concern that some live vaccines can revert to a form that causes more problems.

Investigating inactivated vaccines

Unlike live vaccines, inactivated vaccines are dead. You may wonder what good a dead vaccine is, compared to a live one. The answer is, it's not as good if you really hate injections.

Immunity from inactivated vaccines don't last as long as live vaccines do, so you need more booster shots to keep up your immunity. In some cases, such as the influenza, or flu, vaccine, this is actually a good thing because it allows scientists to change the virus in the vaccine every year to hopefully "match" the type of flu virus that's most prevalent that year.

Contrary to popular opinion, inactivated viruses don't cause the disease they're protecting against. In other words, the flu shot will not give you the flu. However, the flu shot can, like other vaccines, cause a reaction. Typical reactions can include pain at the injection site, muscle aches, and headaches that usually go away in a day or so.

These vaccines don't always create as strong an immune response as a live vaccine. They may need a bit of extra oomph. This can be from an *adjuvant,* a booster that attracts your immune system's attention (as described in Chapter 1). Find out more in Chapter 7.

Other inactivated viruses, such as hepatitis A, rabies, and injectable polio and typhoid vaccines, aren't changed every year like the flu vaccines. For some of these — like injectable typhoid and polio vaccines — you need boosters to keep your immunity up if you'll be exposed to these specific diseases (especially if you're traveling to an area at risk).

Subunit vaccines

Subunit vaccines use only a specific part of the bacteria or virus. They don't use any living components of the bacteria or virus. These are newer vaccines that have been developed as lab technology has advanced. Subunit vaccines first started being used in the 1970s and 1980s. As technology has advanced, new vaccines have become available.

These vaccines use proteins or sugars found in the pathogen that help our immune system recognize the whole pathogen if it ever runs across it. Researchers work hard to find an identifying feature that's really memorable, like a strange tattoo in a "Wanted" photo, which won't change over time. In other words, they pick the germ equivalent of a permanent tattoo rather than a hair color on a "Wanted" poster.

Subunit vaccines don't create as strong an immune response as other types of vaccines and so may need something extra, which is called an adjuvant, to boost the response. These vaccines can protect you against hepatitis B, human papillomavirus (HPV), meningococcal disease, pneumococcal disease, shingles, pertussis or whooping cough, and haemophilus influenzae type b (Hib).

Subunit vaccines can fall into one of the following categories:

>> **Protein-based vaccines,** such as hepatitis B, where a protein that's usually found on the outside of the virus is used alone. This provides enough information for the immune system to remember and later recognize hepatitis B.

>> **Vaccines made from virus-like particles or molecules that look like viruses** but are not infectious because they lack the genetic material, or instructions, to be able to reproduce themselves. These vaccines can occur naturally, or they can be produced in a lab.

>> **Conjugate vaccines** join a protein to an antigen, such as a sugar from the pathogen. This can boost your immune response, where the antigen or sugar alone may not create a strong enough response by itself.

>> **Polysaccharide vaccines,** made up of long chains of sugars that look like the surface of some bacteria, help your immune system respond to the germ in the future.

The conjugate vaccines can be used in small children, but only children age 2 or older have a mature enough immune system to respond to a polysaccharide vaccine. There's a pneumonia vaccine that can be used only after age 2, while a different vaccine can be used for younger children.

Toxoid vaccines

While a toxoid vaccine may not sound like anything you'd want to have injected into your body, these vaccines can be lifesaving. Toxoid vaccines are so named because they take the harmful part of a germ, the toxin that some germs release, and create a vaccine that fights against the harmful germ. A *toxoid* is an inactivated version of the toxin and can't cause the disease it is used to protect against.

These vaccines were first developed in the 1920s, but they work so well that we use similar vaccines today. Their protection doesn't last as long as other vaccines do, so you need boosters to keep your immunity active. Diphtheria and tetanus vaccines are two examples of toxoid vaccine.

Nucleic acid vaccines

Nucleic acid vaccines are a new type of vaccine that are being used to make a strong immune response. *Nucleic acids* are complex compounds found in every living cell. They carry genetic information and are essential for protein synthesis. Before COVID-19, there had never been a nucleic acid vaccine approved in any country, but the first two vaccines to complete Phase III trials and be authorized for use were mRNA (messenger ribonucleic acid, a type of nucleic acid) vaccines. (See Chapter 3 for more on the COVID-19 vaccine.)

These vaccines work by sending in a tiny piece of non-infectious genetic material that tells your body how to produce the protein, the antigen, which will let your body recognize the pathogen in the future. They do not include the whole germ or instructions for the whole germ, so there is no chance of creating the illness. If they're considered "Wanted" pictures, they're like a Snapchat photo that fades and disappears quickly.

REMEMBER

This is the downside of these vaccines; they just don't last very long. They don't last long in our bodies, and they don't last long on the shelf in vials either. To keep them from breaking down and disintegrating (into the basic genetic building blocks we all have), they need to be kept extra cold. Really cold, often down to −80 degrees Celsius, or −112 degrees Fahrenheit, to not break down before being given. Don't worry — they can be warmed up before being given to you!

Viral vector vaccines

Viral vector vaccines use viruses to carry in directions for the "Wanted" picture. They're not made from the virus that we're vaccinating against. They use a simple virus that doesn't make you sick.

They may use a simple cold virus, like an adenovirus or even a modified adenovirus from chimpanzees. In the laboratory, researchers then insert genes into these viruses so that in our bodies they will produce the proteins we need to create an immune response to the target pathogen.

That means the viruses secretly carry in the instructions for the "Wanted" photo for our immune system. We don't want a viral vector to be a virus we already have immunity to, or it may not create much of a response. Ebola vaccines use this technology, as do some COVID-19 vaccines, including the Johnson & Johnson vaccine. The COVID-19 vaccines in use do not make copies of themselves; they use non-replicating viruses.

Testing Vaccines for Safety and Effectiveness

It takes time and a great deal of testing before new vaccines are brought to market. You've probably seen this clearly with the race for development of a vaccine to prevent COVID-19. Even when a vaccine is desperately needed to save the lives of millions, it has to go through a number of tests, called *clinical trials,* to make sure it's both safe for most people to take and also effective against the disease. Most vaccines take ten years to go from lab to us.

In this section, we explain the process behind developing and then manufacturing and marketing a new vaccine.

Determining the need and costs: The preclinical stage

REMEMBER

Before a vaccine is developed and evaluated, there are often two questions asked: "Is it necessary?" and "Is it cost effective?" An enormous number of vaccines never make it past one of these two questions.

For disorders such as the common cold, a proposed vaccine fails in both areas. The common cold is highly annoying, but a vaccine to prevent colds isn't considered all that necessary. It also costs hundreds of millions of dollars to bring a vaccine to market.

It also would be quite hard to make just one vaccine for the cold because there are many different cold viruses. This is why it can seem like you've had the same cold three times in a year. It's not exactly the same cold; it has a different viral make-up from your last cold. Rhinovirus causes around 30 percent of all common colds, but there are nearly 100 types of rhinoviruses, according to the National Institutes of Health. Creating a vaccine for every type of cold would be nearly impossible, although some scientists have tried.

If a new vaccine or treatment seems to meet both the need and the cost effectiveness requirements, it still needs something more: someone interested in developing it. Before any new vaccine or other drug can be tested on people in the United

States, the researchers behind it must apply to the U.S. Food and Drug Administration (FDA) for permission to study an Investigational New Drug, or IND. There will also need to be an ethical review by an Institutional Review Board. Other countries have their own regulations and procedures for bringing new drugs and vaccines to the market.

Most new medications or treatments are animal tested before being tested on humans. They undergo about two years of lab-based testing. Only about 20 percent of vaccines make it through preclinical, laboratory testing to be tested on people.

Phase I

Phase I of the clinical trial is when the vaccine is first tested in people. The vaccine is tested in healthy people, usually about 20–100 participants. The dose is varied to see whether there are differences in side effects.

The objectives are to ensure that the new medication or treatment is safe and to help identify the right dosage. According to the FDA, around 70 percent of new therapeutics move to Phase II.

Phase II

Phase II continues to test healthy people — around a few hundred. The vaccine is given to a wide array of people, including those whose age and health characteristics fit those who would benefit from the vaccine. One dose is given to everyone. The goal is to see whether the immune system shows signs of responding to the vaccine. This phase also looks for short-term side effects.

Approximately 33 percent of all Phase II trials move on to Phase III, where things really get going.

Phase III

Every new treatment, including vaccines, requires a Phase III trial before it can be marketed. A Phase III trial can have thousands of participants. The best way to do a Phase III study is to randomize the volunteer participants into one of several groups. These are called *randomized controlled trials.* For example, people in a vaccine trial may be randomized to one of two groups:

>> People who are given the vaccine.

>> Those who receive a placebo instead of the studied vaccine. They may receive another vaccine, or they may receive an injection of salt water instead.

Participants know they're in one of these two groups but don't know which group they're in. For a clinical trial to give accurate and unbiased results, the groups should be as evenly matched as possible by age, risk factors, and health issues. The study should also be *double-blind*, meaning not only do the participants not know which group they are in, but no one else does either. Researchers only find out at the end, when they unblind the trial.

The goal of Phase III is to determine whether people who receive the vaccine are less likely to develop the disease they are trying to prevent, without causing concerning side effects. Sometimes a participant can become ill or injured during the study. With so many thousands of participants, it's common for this to happen. The illness or injury can be anything, from something that may be related to the vaccine to something unrelated, like being hit by lightning (as actually happened in one COVID-19 trial).

If an unexpected serious adverse event (SAE) occurs, the trial may be paused while the event can be studied independently. The trial is restarted only if it's thought to be safe after this review. These reviews are done by independent committees, called data and safety monitoring boards (DSMB) made up of physicians, statisticians, and other professionals who can pause or end a trial at any point if they have safety concerns. The DSMB can also be involved in Phase I and Phase II to monitor for safety concerns.

As per the FDA, about 25 to 30 percent of pharmaceuticals tested make it past Phase III.

Post-Phase III

After a vaccine has gone through these three phases, there are still more steps before it reaches you. The vaccine needs to be authorized by the FDA, whose approval will be based on an independent review of the data from these trials.

In an emergency, like COVID-19, instead of being FDA approved, the vaccine may have Emergency Use Authorization so that the vaccine can be used more rapidly.

Once the vaccine is approved for use, there will be further monitoring for any side effects and for effectiveness overall. (We discuss this post-authorization monitoring in Chapter 7.)

Studying the Efficacy of Vaccines

Clinical trials take place under controlled circumstances with cherry-picked groups of participants. Participants selected to be in clinical trials are chosen in an attempt to represent the entire population — having a mix of men and women, young and old, different ethnicities and races, and different medical conditions in Phase III trials. Even under these controlled circumstances, however, not everyone who receives the active vaccine will become immune to the disease. The number who do become immune determines the efficacy of the vaccine.

In the following sections, we look at the ways a vaccine's effectiveness is determined, and the difference between efficacy and effectiveness.

Measuring efficacy versus effectiveness

REMEMBER

Efficacy and effectiveness aren't exactly the same thing. Efficacy describes how well the vaccine worked under controlled conditions in a study. Once the vaccine goes into general use, its actual effectiveness is how well it works in the real world:

>> *Vaccine efficacy* is calculated in Phase III (which we discuss earlier in this chapter). Efficacy compares the number of infections among those who get the actual vaccine with the number of infections in the control group who don't receive the vaccine. If a vaccine has 80 percent efficacy, there was an 80 percent reduction in the number of cases in the control group compared with the placebo group. This means that if in a study, 5 percent of the placebo group were infected but 1 percent of the vaccinated group were infected, then the reduction is 80 percent. The vaccine, then, has 80 percent efficacy. Such a vaccine isn't perfect, but it provides a good chance of preventing illness.

>> *Vaccine effectiveness* measures how much illness the vaccine prevents among vaccinated persons in the community. This is usually done by observing differences in the number of illnesses in those who were vaccinated and those who were not vaccinated. There may be reasons in the real world why the vaccine may not work as well; some people may be older or have more medical problems, or the vaccine may not match the strain in the community. There may also be reasons why some people are vaccinated and others are not.

>> *Community effectiveness* measures how much a vaccine prevents disease among everyone in the community. This value compares how much the disease spreads in a community without the vaccine and with the vaccine. As the COVID-19 vaccine has been rolled out, some communities have had

vaccination programs before others. Researchers have studied how well the vaccine protects everyone in the community.

The value is technically this: 1 – ratio of infections in a community with vaccination to infections in a community without vaccinations. This means if 4 percent of the population became infected without a vaccine program and 2 percent did with a vaccine program in place in their community, that the community effectiveness is 1 – $\frac{2}{4}$, or 50 percent. This helps us see herd immunity in real life (see the next section).

Rounding up herd immunity

Herd immunity, also called population immunity, occurs when a large percentage of the community (meaning the "herd") is vaccinated and immune to a disease. This means the disease would be hard to spread if someone were to suddenly arrive with it.

For example, imagine an island and consider the following scenarios:

>> If everyone has been vaccinated with an effective flu vaccine and someone shows up with the flu, that flu isn't going to spread to anyone.

>> If almost everyone has been vaccinated, the person who arrives with the flu is probably not going to bump into anyone who can get sick, but even if they do, those they infect won't easily be able to infect anyone else.

>> If only a few people have been vaccinated, the flu will probably spread from person to person, creating an outbreak.

>> If no one has been vaccinated on the island and no one has had the flu before, then the virus will spread initially unchecked by immunity. How many people are infected and how many need to be vaccinated will depend on a concept called R0 (pronounced R-naught).

REMEMBER

Ro is the number of infections one person will cause if he enters into a group with no immunity. This concept is important because it tells us how many people need to be vaccinated in order to keep a virus from spreading. How effective the vaccine is will also figure in:

>> If R0 is less than 1, then the virus won't be able to continue to spread. That's because there won't be a new infection to replace each infection that recovers (or dies). The virus may cause a few cases, but it will peter out.

>> If R0 is high, like 12 to 18, which we see with measles, a lot more people need to be vaccinated. To stop a measles outbreak from happening, about 93–95 percent need to be vaccinated.

>> If R0 is lower, like an R0 between 1 and 2, which we see with the flu, not as many people need to be vaccinated to stop the virus from spreading.

REMEMBER

Once there is enough immunity in the community so that the virus — or other microbe — doesn't spread, herd immunity is achieved. It's important to have herd immunity. Some people — who are immunocompromised, too young, or pregnant — may not be able to take the vaccine. Vaccines also don't work 100 percent for everyone, so having everyone be protected collectively helps everyone.

Tracing the History of Various Vaccines

Most vaccines these days take about ten years to develop. It takes an incredible investment to design a vaccine and to fully test it for safety. The decision to continue is made at each phase of development.

Past vaccines have all sorts of histories. They were developed by different people in different places at different times. The smallpox vaccine was the first to be used, but others soon followed. Here's a short chronological history of the first vaccines.

Smallpox

Inoculation, also called variolation, to eliminate the scourge of smallpox started as early as the tenth century in China and can actually have been used even earlier. Inoculation or variolation involved taking tiny amounts of material from smallpox lesions and inserting them under the skin of those who were not immune. This led to a mild infection that protected against more serious natural infections. Others developed or practiced inoculation for centuries around the world.

Inoculation was introduced to the United States in 1721 by a man named Onesimus in Boston, Massachusetts, who had been kidnapped into slavery from West Africa. In the same year, inoculation was introduced in England by Mary Montagu, the wife of England's ambassador to what is now Turkey, who found out about the practice in Turkey. Later it was realized that those who had cowpox lesions from working with livestock did not develop smallpox.

Edward Jenner demonstrated the use of the first vaccine in 1796 by first injecting a child with material from a cowpox lesion. When the child had some mild symptoms but no signs of smallpox, Jenner injected material from a fresh smallpox lesion into the boy. This type of clinical trial would never be allowed today! However, this was actually the standard of care at the time for smallpox protection. It was the standard practice to use inoculation to protect the boy as Dr. Jenner did here with smallpox. Luckily, the child didn't develop smallpox after the injection.

Different versions of this vaccine, with a lot more testing, were used over the years until smallpox was eventually eradicated all over the world. This vaccine worked so well that no one in the public needs to be vaccinated for smallpox today.

Typhoid fever

The typhoid vaccine was first developed to help save the lives of soldiers who, at that time, more often died from typhoid than battle. The bacteria that causes typhoid was first identified in 1880. The first vaccine was developed 16 years later. Credit for development of a vaccine belongs to two men: a British pathologist, Sir Almroth Wright, and a German scientist, Richard Pfeiffer. Pfeiffer worked with guinea pigs to find ways to destroy both the typhus and cholera bacteria; Wright developed the actual vaccine.

Untreated typhoid can last for months and kills around 30 percent of its victims. Today, typhoid still affects around 220 million people each year worldwide, and causes around 220,000 deaths. Most occur in areas with poor sanitation, as the bacteria responsible spread via the fecal-oral route.

Yellow fever

Yellow fever was an important virus in the 1800s. One summer in 1793, 10 percent of Philadelphia died from yellow fever. In the following years, the epidemic struck other areas in the United States, like New York and Louisiana. The deadly virus also spread in the Caribbean and in Central and South America. The first vaccine developed against it in the 1920s turned out to be aimed at a different disease, leptospirosis, and didn't work; its developer actually died from yellow fever while trying to correct his mistake and find the right vaccine. Other researchers also died in the quest to make a vaccine that worked.

An early vaccine was developed in the late 1920s. By 1937, a vaccine was developed that was used for a large vaccine campaign. Its discoverer also developed yellow fever while researching the vaccine but survived.

Influenza

Influenza, more commonly called "flu" now, was first identified in 1933, and experimental vaccines were developed soon after around the world. The United States first began vaccinating in 1940.

REMEMBER

Flu vaccines, like the flu itself, are different every year. The vaccine you receive in a given year is a special mix made to match the current circulating strains. The components have to be chosen six months before the flu season so there's enough time to make enough vaccines for everyone who wants the vaccine. The choice in the spring is made based on which strains are most common in the opposite hemisphere — Northern or Southern — where it's autumn and flu season has already begun. Some years the vaccine is more effective than others because the strains circulating may differ from what was expected.

Polio

Polio epidemics in the early 1900s terrified parents and led to public panic as children suddenly became paralyzed, sometimes soon after a swim in a community pool. There was a race to develop an effective vaccine.

An oral, live, attenuated vaccine was used in some parts of the world by 1950. It took until 1952 for the first vaccine to be used in the United States, an injectable vaccine by Jonas Salk and his team. An oral, live, attenuated vaccine from Albert Sabin and his team was licensed in 1961.

Anthrax

The anthrax vaccine was one of the earliest vaccines, developed initially for livestock. The disease was studied throughout much of the 1800s. The bacteria were first identified in 1877, and the first vaccine was made in 1881 for sheep.

A human vaccine was developed in 1950 as farmers were sometimes infected and there was a concern that military troops could be attacked with anthrax.

Measles, mumps, and rubella (MMR)

The MMR vaccine is the combination of the measles, mumps, and rubella vaccines. Measles had been recognized as a problem for centuries, but the first vaccine was licensed in 1963 in the United States. The first mumps and rubella vaccines were licensed in 1967 and 1969, respectively, also in the United States. The vaccines were combined in 1971. Today this vaccine is often given as MMRV with varicella (or chicken pox) added as well; see the next section for more about varicella.

Varicella (chicken pox)

Varicella zoster, the virus that causes chicken pox, has been known as a disease separate from smallpox since the late 18th century. Work on varicella vaccines began in the 1920s. The first effective chicken pox vaccine to be licensed was developed in 1974 for children with immune system issues, such as leukemia. It wasn't used in the general population until 1986, first in Japan in the 1970s. It was licensed in the United States in 1995.

The chicken pox vaccine still isn't used everywhere in the world, and its use is only targeted (such as for exposed healthcare workers) in the United Kingdom.

Chapter **6**

Tracking the Current List of Effective Vaccines

When you're a kid, it seems like every other month you're at the doctor's office getting an injection. And then you become an adult, and it seems like you need to have more and more vaccines. Yes, there are a lot of vaccines, and yes, you really do benefit from every last one in most cases. In this chapter, we describe the current vaccines, explain how they work, and focus on their purpose and their effectiveness. (For an in-depth look at the newest vaccines — the COVID-19 vaccines — turn to Chapter 3.)

Chicken Pox (Varicella)

If you're over age 40 or so, you may have a vivid memory of chicken pox, also called *varicella*. Having endured the itchiness and temporarily miserable feeling and lived to tell the tale, you may question why a vaccine against such a mild disease even exists. The answer is that while chicken pox is generally annoying but harmless in the long run for most people, in a rare few, chicken pox can be deadly. Chicken pox is extremely contagious, with an R0 of around 10, which means that each person who develops chicken pox usually infects around 10 other people who aren't immune. (*R0* is the number of people infected by one sick person. It's a way of describing how contagious a disease is.)

Of the four million people who got chicken pox each year in the United States before the vaccine was widely given starting in 1995, around 100 to 150 people died from chicken pox each year and between 10,000 to 13,000 people were hospitalized. Complications from chicken pox include infections such as pneumonia and *encephalitis*, a brain infection. It also causes parents to miss work and children to miss school. The vaccine also reduces the chance of having shingles later on (we cover the shingles vaccine later in this chapter). Since 1995, the incidence of deaths from chicken pox has decreased by 94 percent.

The chicken pox vaccine is a live attenuated vaccine. (See Chapter 5 for info on different types of vaccines.) The vaccine is generally given to young children to prevent them from catching the disease early on. (See Chapters 8 and 9 for more on vaccination schedules.)

WARNING

Because the vaccine is made from the live virus, people with weakened immune systems shouldn't get it. Pregnant women and people who are allergic to ingredients used to make the vaccine should also not take it. Because chicken pox can be dangerous in pregnancy, it's important to be immune or vaccinated before pregnancy.

Side effects of the vaccine can include a sore arm at the site of the shot, a mild fever, a rash at the site of the shot, temporary joint pain, or achiness. More serious complications include allergic reactions such as hives or trouble breathing.

Two chicken pox vaccines are licensed for use in the United States: Varivax, which provides immunity only to chicken pox, and MMRV (brand name ProQuad in the United States), which provides immunity to chicken pox as well as measles, mumps, and rubella. We talk about the MMRV vaccine later in this chapter.

Diphtheria, Tetanus, and Pertussis

Diphtheria, tetanus, and pertussis are three very different infections that we vaccinate for all together. They are given in infancy and up to age 7 as the DTaP vaccine and as the Tdap in adults and children over 7. Thanks to this combined vaccine, diphtheria and tetanus, which both used to cause a lot of suffering, are rarely seen in the United States and much less common worldwide.

Diphtheria

Diphtheria was once called the "Strangling Angel" of children. It's a horrible disease that killed as many as one in five kids who got sick. It can cause thick secretions, called *pseudomembranes*, that clog the throat, making it harder and harder to breathe. It's awful to see and is the reason intubation was first invented in the 1800s in a desperate attempt to save these children.

The disease is due to the toxins produced by bacteria called *Corynebacterium diphtheriae*. It can cause a fever, a sore throat, and heart problems, as well as kidney and nerve problems. Before antibiotics and vaccines were available, horses were used to create antitoxins, or antibodies, for this bacteria, and these antitoxins are still used today when unvaccinated children become sick.

The diphtheria vaccine, a killed vaccine, was developed in the 1920s. (Chapter 5 gives a more detailed explanation of the vaccine's history.) Before the 1980s, it was thought there were a million cases a year worldwide; now there are fewer than 20,000 a year reported globally.

In the 1940s, the diphtheria vaccine was combined with tetanus and pertussis vaccines, two other killed vaccines.

Tetanus

Tetanus is more than just the if-you-step-on-a-rusty-nail shot. In fact, the rust on the nail isn't why you need an up-to-date tetanus shot at all. It's the Clostridium bacteria *(Clostridium tetani)*, found in soil as well as saliva, manure, and even on skin and dust. A rusty nail, a cut, a dirty injection, or a burn can let the bacteria get deep into the wound.

Tetanus causes muscles to spasm. This can be mild in some, but it can also make it hard to breathe, requiring intubation. It's known for causing a "sardonic smile" as muscles lock up and force an uncomfortable smile. It also causes lockjaw and makes it hard to open the jaw and eat. Deaths from tetanus dropped 99 percent in the United States after the vaccine was introduced in the 1940s. Tetanus antitoxins can come from horses, but human and lab-made antibodies are also used to treat this infection if someone who is not vaccinated becomes sick.

REMEMBER

The vaccine is made from tetanus toxoid, which is a gentle version of the toxin the bacteria produces but modified (by heat or chemicals, like formalin) to cause no harm. Our immune systems can be trained to recognize the toxin from exposure to the toxoid. If you ever have a dirty wound, burn, or puncture wound that can be a source of tetanus, it's important to have a repeat vaccine if you haven't finished your childhood boosters or haven't had a shot in five years. After infancy and childhood boosters, further boosters are recommended every ten years, since immunity decreases over time.

Pertussis

Pertussis, or whooping cough, causes just what it sounds like — uncontrollable coughing spells. The cough can sound like a seal barking. This disease can be a troublesome cough for adults, but it can be deadly for children, especially infants, who are too young to be vaccinated and may catch the bacteria from a visiting relative.

The first vaccine, developed in 1914 and combined in 1948 with the tetanus and diphtheria vaccines, dropped the rate of disease from the 100,000s to little more than 1,000 to 4,000 cases each year. Earlier versions of the vaccine were not as effective at controlling outbreaks and also had some side effects.

A new vaccine was developed in the 1990s that was better tolerated and created a better immune response, using material from part of the cell rather than the whole cell. The current vaccines have an "a" to show they have a cell-free (or *acellular*) vaccine make-up. They're known as Tdap or DTaP to indicate the acellular material used. DTaP can also be given as the DTaP-Inactivated Polio Vaccine, or the DTaP-IPV/Hib (haemophilus influenzae type b) combined vaccine (see the next section). Sometimes tetanus and diphtheria vaccines are given alone without pertussis.

Haemophilus Influenzae Type B (Hib)

The vaccine against this germ, which sounds like a virus but is actually a bacteria called *Haemophilus influenzae type b* (Hib), is a relative newcomer. This vaccine can be given alone or in combination with other vaccines as the DTaP-IPV/Hib vaccine (see the previous section for more on DTaP, otherwise known as diphtheria, tetanus, and pertussis). Hib can cause pneumonia, a bloodstream infection, an infection of the epiglottis (which protects the windpipe; the disease makes it hard to breathe), and meningitis (an inflammation of the meninges, which surround the brain and spinal cord). This infection usually affects those under age 5, but some adults are also at risk.

Before the vaccine was developed, Hib was the leading cause of bacterial meningitis in children under 5 in the United States, and around 1,000 of those children died from the infection each year. Around 20 percent of children who had Hib meningitis had hearing loss or other long-term neurologic or nerve damage. It used to be common for pediatric wings of the hospital to fill up with children battling this infection. The vaccine, developed in the early 1990s, decreased the incidence of Hib by 99 percent. Collectively, the use of the vaccine has made this infection a rarity.

The Hib vaccine is a type of inactivated bacterial vaccine that uses just a part of the bacteria. It is specifically a polysaccharide conjugate vaccine, where a piece of the polysaccharide outer layer of the bacteria is attached to a protein that acts as the carrier.

It's given as a series of injections in young children, either alone or in combination with other vaccines, such as the DTaP-IPV vaccine. This vaccine is important not only for young children but also for people who do not have a spleen due to injury, surgery, or sickle cell disease. The vaccine should not be taken by those who have had a severe allergy to the ingredients in the vaccines or who are under 6 weeks old. The course is either two or three doses and generally protects up to 95 percent of children. Typical side effects, such as fever, redness, or swelling at the site, can occur after vaccination.

Hepatitis A

Hepatitis viruses affect the liver, one of the most important organs in your body, with over 500 essential tasks to keep your body working optimally. Hepatitis A virus is the most common type of the five hepatitis viruses: A, B, C, D, and E. Vaccines protect only against types A and B at present (see the next section for details on the hepatitis B vaccine). Most countries use an inactivated vaccine, so there's no chance that you'll get the disease from the vaccine.

The vaccine for hepatitis A first became available in 1995. Hepatitis A can be spread through food or drink or through person-to-person contact. Examples include the following:

>> It can spread from raw shellfish, especially oysters, as well as raw fruits and vegetables.

>> It can be transmitted by someone who doesn't wash their hands and then touches your food. Outbreaks can be triggered at a restaurant if a food handler is infected.

>> The virus can come from drinking water contaminated with sewage.

>> It can spread when a day-care worker changes the diaper of a child who is sick.

Unlike hepatitis B and C, hepatitis A infection usually lasts just a short time. But a short time can be up to several months, and in rare cases, hepatitis A can be fatal. Symptoms of hepatitis A can include fever, tiredness, stomach pain, diarrhea or vomiting, a yellow tinge to the whites of the eyes or under the tongue, dark urine, or light-colored stools.

The hepatitis vaccine is given in a series of two shots six months apart. Both injections are necessary to provide immunity in most cases. Children between 12 and 23 months are usually given the injections, as are older children who missed the initial vaccines.

TIP

A combination vaccine that provides protection against hepatitis A and B can be given to adults in a series of three shots within six months. There's also a combination hepatitis A and typhoid vaccine that can provide protection against both of these diseases.

Your doctor may recommend the hepatitis A vaccine if you

>> Have been exposed to someone with hepatitis A

>> Are traveling internationally

>> Are experiencing homelessness

>> Are a child or an adolescent

>> Will have close contact with an international adoptee

>> Are a man who has sex with men

>> Engage in any type of drug use

>> Have chronic liver disease

>> Have HIV or another immunosuppressive disorder

>> Have an occupational risk (such as a sewage worker, a childcare employee who has contact with diapers, a food handler in a hospital, and so on)

The vaccine is usually protective against the virus within two to four weeks. The vaccine may provide protection for at least 20 years.

Hepatitis B

The hepatitis B vaccine became available in 1982. Unlike hepatitis A (see the previous section), hepatitis B can cause long-term infection that can damage your liver over years. This occurs in just 2 to 6 percent of adults who are infected with hepatitis B, but it can progress to the point where you may need a liver transplant to survive. Over 800,000 people in the United States live with hepatitis B, with over 20,000 new infections occurring each year.

Infants infected with hepatitis B have a much higher chance of permanent damage than adults who are newly infected; around 90 percent of those infected at birth have serious liver problems. Of adults who are infected, only 2 to 6 percent develop chronic infection. Hepatitis B infection is also the most common cause of liver cancer.

Hepatitis B is passed through blood and is sexually transmitted. It can also be transmitted through needlesticks; sharing needles, razors, or toothbrushes (with potential blood exposure); or contact with open sores or wounds. Pregnant women can also pass the infection to their babies at birth.

Vaccines against hepatitis B are given in infancy via a series of three shots. (See Chapter 8 for more on infant vaccine schedules.) Vaccination is especially important for babies born to mothers with hepatitis B. Two or three injections, depending on the specific vaccine, can protect adults who haven't had the vaccine.

The vaccine is recommended for all infants and children. You should also have the vaccine if

>> Your sexual partner or another family member has hepatitis B

>> You're sexually active and not monogamous

>> You share needles with another person

>> You're a man who has sex with men

>> You're a healthcare worker with potential exposure to blood or other bodily fluids

>> You work or live in a group home for the developmentally disabled

>> You travel to areas where hepatitis B is prevalent

>> You need or may need dialysis

>> You have hepatitis C or another chronic liver disease or HIV

>> You want the vaccine to protect yourself

People who spend time in crowded quarters, such as prison, should also have the vaccine.

The hepatitis B vaccine, like the hepatitis A vaccine, is an inactivated vaccine. Common side effects are soreness or redness at the injection site in the arm.

Human Papillomavirus (HPV)

Human papillomaviruses, or HPVs, include over 200 viruses, of which 40 can be sexually transmitted. Others can spread by direct skin contact. Most people get some form of this virus. HPV can affect both men and women, and it's the most common cause of sexually transmitted infection in the United States. HPV infections can lead to cervical cancer, which used to be the leading cause of cancer worldwide, but thanks to Pap smears and the vaccines, it is now the fourth worldwide and eighth in the United States. HPVs can also cause anal, penile, vaginal, and vulvar cancers. Up to 70 percent of all oropharyngeal cancers may also be related to HPV. HPV can also cause genital warts, which can be transmitted to a newborn during the passage through the birth canal.

Vaccines against HPVs became available in the United States in 2006. The U.S. vaccine, Gardisil 9, protects against nine types of HPV, including types 16 and 18, which cause 70 percent of all cervical cancers. It also protects against types 6 and 11, which cause up to 90 percent of genital warts. In addition, Gardisil 9 provides immunity to five other HPVs — types 31, 33, 45, 52, and 58 — which together cause between 10 and 20 percent of cervical cancers.

The HPV vaccine uses virus-like particles (VLPs) found on the surface of the virus to provide immunity. The VLPs contain no DNA and can't cause an infection. Typical side effects include pain, redness or swelling at the injection site on the arm, fever, dizziness or fainting, muscle or joint pain, fatigue, nausea, or headache.

HPV vaccines should be given to boys and girls starting at age 11. By age 15, around 10 percent of girls already have HPV infection, and this rises to nearly 20 percent by age 17.

TECHNICAL STUFF

In 2021, just two states — Virginia and Rhode Island — and Washington, DC, require the vaccine for school attendance. Parents can opt out for medical, moral, or religious reasons.

People given the vaccine before age 15 need two injections; those who begin the series after this age need three injections to provide immunity. HPV vaccines won't cure a current HPV infection. The vaccine is not recommended during pregnancy, but if given, because it's not a live vaccine, it is not expected to be associated with any risk and none has been identified. Protection appears to last at least 10 years. Researchers are still following to see how long it provides protection.

Influenza (Flu)

REMEMBER

Unlike most other vaccines, the flu vaccine needs to be updated each year. You need to hold out your arm for another jab every year if you want to reduce your risk of flu.

Despite the availability of the flu vaccine, between 10 and 49 million people in the United States, or between 20 percent and 50 percent of the population, get the flu each year. The flu vaccine, while not perfect, reduces the chance of getting the flu by 40 to 60 percent. Its effectiveness can depend on how well the vaccine matches the strains spreading that year. But only around 50 percent of Americans get a flu vaccine every year.

Part of the reason for the reduced effectiveness of the flu vaccine is that the flu changes from year to year. There are three types of influenza virus — A, B, and C — that affect humans (see Chapter 2 for details). Influenza A and B, and their numerous subtypes, cause most of the flu illnesses (see the nearby sidebar "Naming each year's flu" for more about the make-up of flu viruses and vaccines). So each year, the world has to determine which flu subtypes are likely to spread. This is done in the Northern Hemisphere by looking six months ahead at the Southern Hemisphere's flu make-up as a guide to the next year's fall and winter viruses.

Most years' flu vaccines contain influenza A (H1N1) and influenza A (H3N2) — the two most common types of influenza virus — and one or two influenza B viruses.

Flu vaccines were first developed in the 1930s but weren't in widespread use until 1945, when it was approved for the military and then for civilians. Many vaccines have been developed or initially distributed by the military to keep troops safe.

There are several types of injectable and inactivated flu vaccines, including the following:

>> Injectable flu vaccines that use inactivated materials and were originally grown using fertilized chicken eggs

>> Newer injected vaccines that use mammalian cells rather than eggs to produce the vaccines (Flucelvax)

>> Recombinant vaccines, which use DNA from a cell on the influenza virus and a different virus, called a *baculovirus,* to produce the hemagglutinin antigen that stimulates antibody production (Flublok)

NAMING EACH YEAR'S FLU

Every year different flu viruses are prevalent, so the science of producing a vaccine that protects against the most likely flu bug candidates for the following year is complex. Sometimes scientists pick the wrong viruses, and the flu vaccine ends up being not very effective against that year's circulating strains.

Influenza A and B cause most cases of flu. Type A has two subtypes, named for the proteins on their surfaces, hemagglutinin (H) and neuraminidase (N). The subtypes are further broken down into groups; the H group has 18 subgroups, and N has 11. So the 2009 swine flu epidemic, called H1N1, was an influenza A with subtypes H1 and N1.

Altogether, the various types of H and N can combine to make 198 types of influenza A, although only 131 have been found to occur. To confuse things even more, the two subtypes are further divided into groups, or *clades,* which are subdivided again into subgroups or sub-clades.

The most common current circulating A viruses are H1N1 and H3N2. The whole names may be written like so:

- A/Victoria/2570/2019 (H1N1)pdm09-like virus

- A/Cambodia/e0826360/2020 (H3N2)-like virus

The "pdm09" represents pandemic 2009, as the descendants of the 2009 H1N1 pandemic continue to spread.

These two viruses are included in the 2021–2022 Northern Hemisphere vaccine.

Type B influenza variants are named after lineages — which are specifically B/Yamagata and B/Victoria; B viruses change more slowly from year to year than type A influenza viruses. The two variants can also be subdivided into clades.

Influenza subtypes are also named after the animal host in which they first appeared, if it wasn't from a human subtype. The area where the virus first originated can also be part of its official name, as well as the year when it first appeared and its strain.

For instance, the two influenza B choices for the 2021–2022 Northern Hemisphere vaccine are

- B/Washington/02/2019 (B/Victoria lineage)-like virus

- B/Phuket/3073/2013 (B/Yamagata lineage)-like virus

The nasal spray flu vaccine uses a live attenuated virus to produce antibodies. For adults over 65, there are vaccines with higher doses or that contain an *adjuvant,* a substance that helps create a stronger immune reaction. The flu vaccine can be given to children over age 6 months. It's also safe and important for pregnant women to have a flu shot, as the flu can be a terrible infection in pregnancy, but pregnant women should avoid the nasal live vaccine.

Measles, Mumps, and Rubella (MMR)

Measles, mumps, and rubella, also called German measles, are three common childhood diseases that can have devastating consequences. In the 1970s, vaccines against all three were combined in a single injection called the MMR vaccine. The MMR vaccine is a live attenuated vaccine, so there is a live but harmless virus in the vaccine. Two doses of the MMR vaccine provide immunity in 97 percent of people from measles and rubella and 88 percent against mumps.

Here are a few details about each disease:

>> **Measles** causes a rash, high fever, cough, runny nose, and pink eye. It's also extremely contagious and, in some cases, fatal. Pneumonia and encephalitis, a brain infection, can also follow measles. (See Chapter 2 for more about the measles vaccine and its development.)

>> **Mumps** causes swelling of the parotid or saliva glands, which gives a characteristic "chipmunk" look. Headache, low-grade fever, and tiredness can also accompany mumps. But more seriously, mumps can also cause a testicular infection called *orchitis* in as many as one-third of males, which can lead to infertility. And, until the vaccine was developed in 1967, mumps was the most common cause of meningitis and acquired deafness in children in the United States.

TECHNICAL STUFF

The mumps vaccine was the quickest ever brought to market at that time, though much earlier vaccines, like the typhoid vaccine in 1896, as well as rabies and smallpox vaccines, were used right after they were developed. It became available in four years, and the scientist instrumental in its development was spurred on by his own daughter's case of the mumps. He named the mumps strain used to make the vaccine after his daughter, Jeryl Lynn, whose throat he cultured the strain from. This strain was used to make a live attenuated vaccine, which replaced a killed vaccine in 1978 and is still used today.

>> **Rubella** can cause serious problems during pregnancy to the unborn fetus. Symptoms are generally mild in children and adults, and they include a rash that starts on the face and then spreads. Other symptoms include a low-grade fever, possible headache, sore throat, and general fatigue. A fetus may die in utero or develop serious birth defects if mom catches rubella during her pregnancy. In the last major outbreak in the United States, around 12 million people, mostly children, had rubella. The vaccine has eliminated rubella in the United States since 2004, although it still exists in other countries.

The first dose of MMR vaccine is given between the ages of 12 and 15 months, and the second dose is administered between ages 4 and 6. The first dose may be given earlier if there is an outbreak, but in these cases two doses are still required at age 12 months and older. The vaccine is not as effective under 12 months, in part because of leftover antibodies from mom and the baby's young immune system, but giving the vaccine early isn't harmful.

Around 4 in 10,000 children have a febrile seizure after this injection. While frightening, there are no known long-term effects from this.

Adults born before 1957 are presumed to be immune from these diseases, which were widely spread before vaccines were developed. However, if you work in healthcare and do not have documented antibodies, you should have the vaccine. Adults born after this time may require two injections of the vaccine to provide immunity if they haven't had these diseases. You may need to wait to have the MMR vaccine. You should talk to your doctor about whether you should have the MMR vaccine now if any of the following apply:

>> You have an allergic reaction to a prior vaccination or any component of this vaccine (including gelatin, neomycin).

>> You're pregnant.

>> You have immune issues, such as untreated AIDS; you take meds that weaken your immune system; you have leukemia; or you are concerned you may have an immune issue. Talk to your doctor, but you can have this vaccine if you have HIV, but not AIDS.

>> You've had another vaccine within the last few weeks. Live vaccines given too close together can weaken the effects of the vaccine.

>> You have had a blood transfusion or other blood products within the past three months.

>> You have had low platelets or thrombocytopenia.

>> You're feeling ill.

As always, talk to your doctor before receiving any vaccine.

Measles, Mumps, Rubella, and Varicella (MMRV)

The measles, mumps, rubella, and varicella vaccine adds the varicella, or chicken pox, vaccine to the MMR mix. This vaccine is given only to children aged 12 months to 12 years and was first marketed in 2005. We cover both varicella and MMR earlier in this chapter.

The MMRV vaccine can cause side effects similar to other vaccines, including a sore arm, redness at the injection site, and a low-grade fever and/or rash. In rare cases, seizure can occur after the vaccine; this occurs about twice as often after the MMRV vaccine as it does when the MMR and varicella vaccines are given separately. Although this worries parents, it causes no long-term damage. Also rarely, fever and rash can occur up to 42 days after the injection.

Meningococcal Vaccines

Meningitis — a viral or bacterial infection that affects the *meninges*, the membranes that line the brain and spinal cord — can cause numerous serious and sometimes permanent health problems. These infections can also cause death. Meningitis spreads easily in crowded places such as colleges, military installations, or prisons. Sometimes there can be outbreaks on college campuses, which make the news and can cause deaths in young adults.

Vaccines protect against bacterial infections caused by *Neisseria meningitidis*. Meningitis caused by *Neisseria* bacteria can result in rapid illness that's fatal in about 10 percent of cases. The bacteria that cause meningitis can be carried in the nose and throat by people who aren't sick. Up to 10 to 20 percent of teens and adults carry the bacteria without becoming ill themselves. Even though vaccines are routinely available, between 1,400 and 2,800 cases of meningococcal disease occur each year in the United States. Despite antibiotics, 10 to 15 percent with meningitis die.

Symptoms include fever, headache, stiff neck, confusion, light sensitivity, and nausea. Infants may have a high-pitched cry and be unusually irritable or sleepy; the *fontanelle,* or soft spot on the top of a baby's head, may bulge outward. If the disease progresses to cause blood infection, or *sepsis,* a rash, often with small red dots or purple or red patches that don't fade when pressed, cold hands and feet, and severe muscle and body aches can occur in addition to other symptoms. Up to 20 percent of survivors have long-term side effects, such as brain damage, loss of limbs, or hearing loss.

WARNING

Symptoms of bacterial meningitis occur and progress very rapidly; adults can die within 24 hours and children in even less time. Having bacterial meningitis once does not protect you from getting it again.

Current meningococcal vaccines protect against five strains of *Neisseria meningitidis.* None of the vaccines used contain live material. A *conjugate* vaccine — which combines a weak antigen with a protein for better protection — called MenACWY, or MCV4, gives immunity to the A, C, W, and Y serogroups, the most common causes of meningococcal disease. This vaccine is routinely given to children starting at age 11, with a booster at age 16, and was first approved in 2005. The MenB vaccine gives immunity to the B strain, which occurs less often; this vaccine isn't given routinely but may be given to susceptible individuals, especially in outbreaks, as has occurred on university campuses or in some parts of the world where it is more common, such as seen in Norway, Cuba, and New Zealand.

Pneumococcal Vaccines

Streptococcus pneumoniae is another type of bacteria with numerous serotypes. Like meningococcal bacteria (see the previous section), *S. pneumoniae* or Strep pneumo as it is abbreviated, is found in the nose and throats of healthy people. Children are most likely to carry the bacteria, and as many as one in two may, though it varies. Adults can also be carriers of Strep pneumo, but usually less than 1 in 20 are at any time. The bacteria cause illness when they spread beyond these areas to the lungs or oropharynx.

Strep pneumo most commonly can cause pneumonia, meningitis, ear infections, and *septicemia* (infection in the blood). Pneumococcal bacteria cause 50 percent of all cases of bacterial meningitis. Pneumococcal pneumonia hospitalizes around 150,000 Americans each year and kills between 3,000 and 4,000. Young children and people over age 65 are at greatest risk.

There are a lot of different types of Strep pneumo. Over 90 serotypes are known, making it a bit hard to make a vaccine for each one. The first vaccine was a polysaccharide vaccine licensed in 1977 for 14 types. It was replaced in the 1980s with a polysaccharide vaccine for 23 different types (PPSV23, or Pneumovax 23). A conjugated vaccine was introduced in 2000. The current pneumococcal conjugate vaccine (PCV13 or Prevnar 13) includes the sugars of 13 serotypes of *Streptococcus pneumoniae* attached (or conjugated to) a nontoxic diphtheria toxin in order to get an immune response.

About 80 percent of adults have an immune response to the PPSV23 vaccine, but some with immune issues or who are older do not have as strong a response. It helps that children and others are vaccinated as it reduces transmission to them.

Adults and children receive different vaccines against these bacteria. The main differences are as follows:

» The vaccine given in childhood, Prevnar 13, protects against 13 different serotypes.

» The vaccine for adults, Pneumovax 23, protects against 23 different serotypes.

» The adult vaccine isn't effective in children under age 2.

» One injection is generally sufficient in adults; children require a series of injections.

As with any vaccine, side effects can occur. Most are garden-variety side effects seen with most injections: redness, pain or swelling at the injection site, tiredness, low-grade fever, fussiness, or loss of appetite.

REMEMBER

This vaccine should be given at a different time than some vaccines. You shouldn't have both PCV13 and PPSV23 at the same time; if given both, you should have PCV13 first and then PPSV23 later on. Young children shouldn't have the meningococcal and pneumococcal conjugate vaccines at the same time in order to achieve the best immune response.

The following sections provide more details on the vaccines for adults and for kids.

For adults

In 2019, the recommendations for pneumococcal vaccines for adults changed. The Centers for Disease Control (CDC) no longer routinely recommend both Prevnar 13 and Pneumovax 23 vaccines for adults over age 65; only Pneumovax 23 is routinely given.

Adults with certain health conditions may need to get both vaccines, even if they're under age 65. Both vaccines are recommended if you're at risk for serious pneumococcal complications. Conditions that may require both vaccines in adults include

>> Cancers of the blood, such as leukemia, lymphoma, or multiple myeloma

>> Cancer that's spread beyond the original site (metastatic cancer)

>> Cerebrospinal fluid leakage

>> HIV

>> Immune deficiencies

>> Kidney disease

>> Liver disease

>> Organ transplantation

>> Sickle cell anemia

>> Asplenia, or lack of a spleen

The vaccines can be given about eight weeks apart; Prevnar 13 is best given first. For adults over age 65 who need both vaccines, they're usually given about a year apart. Medicare won't pay for the second vaccine unless they're given at least 11 months apart.

It's also important that the PPSV23 is given to those adults at risk. This includes a broad category of people, including smokers as well as those who have

>> Diabetes

>> Chronic heart or liver disease

>> Alcoholism

>> Asthma

>> Chronic lung disease, including obstructive pulmonary disease

For children

The first pneumococcal vaccine for children protected them against seven serotypes of *S. pneumoniae*; the current vaccine is active against 13. This vaccine provides immunity to over 95 percent of vaccinated children.

Children shouldn't take the vaccine if

>> They're moderately ill at the time of injection

>> They've had a severe allergic reaction to an earlier vaccine dose or to the DTaP vaccine that we discuss earlier in this chapter (as the diphtheria toxin is in the conjugate vaccine).

Let your doctor know if your child runs a high fever or has a serious allergic reaction after an injection.

Rotavirus

The rotavirus vaccine, another relative newcomer to the vaccine family, came into widespread use in 2008. Rotavirus was the main cause of severe diarrhea in children until this vaccine came along. The virus causes gastrointestinal symptoms such as watery diarrhea, abdominal pain, and vomiting, along with fever. There are different serotypes of rotavirus. You can get rotavirus more than once, but after the first time, subsequent bouts are less severe. Children have the highest risk of becoming extremely ill from rotavirus. Symptoms often follow a certain pattern:

>> Fever, stomach pain, and vomiting start first and last several days.

>> Diarrhea starts after the first symptoms subside and can last up to a week.

Before the vaccine, rotavirus was the leading cause of severe diarrhea in infants and younger children, sending between 55,000 and 70,000 to the hospital in the United States, and killing 20 to 40 children each year.

Like many GI infections, rotavirus is passed via the fecal-oral route, making it easily spread in places like day-care centers. The main risk from rotavirus is dehydration, which can be life-threatening in children. Symptoms of dehydration in children include

>> Decreased urination

>> Lack of tears

>> Dry mouth

>> Lethargy

>> In infants, a sunken fontanelle, or soft spot on the top of the head

The rotavirus vaccine is a live attenuated vaccine; four versions are in use worldwide at this time, two of which are used in the United States. Rotavirus vaccination is given by putting drops of the vaccine in the child's mouth. No needles are required. The child needs to return for a total of either two or three doses depending on the manufacturer. The child should complete all the doses before age 8 months. In healthy children, the rotavirus vaccine can be given at the same time as other vaccines.

TECHNICAL STUFF

An earlier vaccine was made available and then withdrawn in 1998 and 1999. It was taken off the market in the 1980s because of a slightly increased risk of *intussusception,* a condition in which the bowel can fold up into the section before it and become blocked. There are other causes of intussusception, and infants can be prone to this with or without being vaccinated.

If your child has a severely weakened immune system, has an allergic reaction, or has had intussusception, your doctor may recommend against the vaccine. In rare cases, the shedding in stool from this live attenuated vaccine can infect others.

Shingles (Herpes Zoster)

Ask anyone who's had shingles and prepare to listen to a tale of pain. Shingles, also called herpes zoster, is caused by the same virus that causes chicken pox, or varicella (covered earlier in this chapter). If you had chicken pox as a child, as 99 percent of people worldwide over age 50 have, the virus hangs around for decades, hiding in the nerve cells of your skin. In around one-third of adults, the virus reactivates at some point, and the painful shingles rash appears.

Shingles causes small blistery bumps that resemble chicken pox to break out along nerve lines. They can occur just about anywhere on your body, and they appear in a line or a cluster. They usually affect just one side of the body at a time. The lesions can be exquisitely painful rather than itchy. The blisters normally develop scabs within seven to ten days and disappear completely within two to four weeks. In addition to the rash, you may also have a headache, fever, and body aches.

In 10 to 13 percent of cases, a condition called post herpetic neuralgia, or PHN, can occur. In PHN, pain along the nerve continues more than 90 days after the infection. The older you are when you have shingles, the more likely you are to develop PHN. Also, if you have shingles around your eye, it can permanently affect your vision.

Usually this rash occurs only in a small section on one side of your body, where the skin is supplied from just one spinal nerve root. If a larger area is affected, more nerves may be involved. This is called disseminated zoster and is more common in those with weakened immune systems, such as from HIV.

Other potential complications include

>> Brain inflammation, also called encephalitis

>> Hearing issues

>> Vision issues

The CDC recommends that adults over age 50 get the shingles vaccine, which is given in two injections two to six months apart. However, only around 35 percent of people over age 60 have had the vaccine.

An earlier vaccine was developed in 2006 called Zostavax and was an attenuated vaccine. Shingrix, a recombinant vaccine that has no live virus, is around 97 percent effective against the virus, which normally affects around one million Americans per year. Shingrix was approved by the Food and Drug Administration (FDA) in 2017. Because it's not a live vaccine, it is probably safe if you have immune system issues, and it has no upper age limit. The older vaccine, Zostavax, a live vaccine, was not recommended for immunosuppressed people or those who have had an organ transplant. Zostavax is no longer used in the United States.

WARNING

You should not have the shingles vaccine if

>> You've had a severe reaction to the vaccine or any of its ingredients

>> You've never had chicken pox (the chicken pox vaccine is recommended instead)

>> You currently have shingles

>> You're pregnant or breastfeeding (as it hasn't been studied in this population)

The shingles vaccine, like most vaccines, can cause minor side effects, such as soreness, redness, or swelling at the injection site. However, it is considered a reactogenic vaccine, so you're more likely to have side effects for a short time as your immune system responds to this vaccine. Fever, fatigue, headache, nausea, or stomach pain can also occur. More serious side effects such as hives, difficulty breathing, or anaphylaxis require immediate medical care.

SAYING GOODBYE TO THE SMALLPOX VACCINE

Thanks to the smallpox vaccine, this disease has been erased from the face of the earth. The last known natural case occurred in 1977 in Somalia, and the last case occurred from a lab accident in the United Kingdom in 1978. Smallpox was declared eradicated in 1979.

The story of the smallpox vaccine is a success story beyond any other. Once a scourge across the world, killing 30 percent of its victims and maiming many of the survivors, smallpox has become just a footnote in history. Inoculations were used with varying success before the smallpox vaccine took the form that finally eliminated the disease altogether. (See Chapter 2 for more on the history of smallpox and the vaccine.) The most recent vaccines used vaccinia, a virus that belongs to the same genus as the smallpox virus.

The last vaccines used against smallpox were live vaccines that presented some serious potential complications. In addition to the pustule that formed at the injection site, which caused noticeable scarring, smallpox vaccines caused typical symptoms such as fever, swollen lymph glands, fatigue, and rash. The material inside the vaccine can, if inadvertently spread to the eyes, mouth, nose, or genitalia, cause lesions in those areas also. Complications such as encephalitis, a rash with eczema, or bloodborne vaccinia, as well as rarely death, can also occur.

The last smallpox vaccines caused more complications than many of the newer vaccines used today for other illnesses. Research on smallpox vaccines made from recombinant DNA may make smallpox vaccination safer if the need for it ever arises again.

Chapter **7**

What to Expect When You're Vaccinating

While vaccine side effects do occur, they're mostly more of a nuisance than a serious problem. Some side effects are common. Others are less common and specific to certain vaccines. Rarely, some side effects can pose a serious health risk. In this chapter, you get the scoop on common side effects, serious reactions, and the effect of many vaccines on the immune system.

REMEMBER

Sometimes what seems like a side effect is actually just an unrelated health problem. Vaccines protect us from specific diseases but don't protect us from everything out there. We can still have new health problems. This is especially true when vaccinating those who are elderly or very young as well as those with weakened immune systems. Sometimes we can just have bad luck after being vaccinated. In one of the COVID-19 vaccine trials, one adverse event that occurred after vaccination was that someone was hit by lightning. No one thinks the vaccine caused that.

Understanding Side Effects: What May Cause Them and What Happens

Over 1 billion vaccines are given worldwide each year. For most people, the side effects are minimal and the benefits have been life-saving. But sometimes your immune system reacts when it sees something new, and this reaction can cause you to have side effects. In some cases, this is a good thing; it shows your immune system is working well.

You *should* react in some way to a foreign object in your body. In the same way that your skin might turn red or irritated around a splinter, your arm can react to an injection with common symptoms, such as redness or swelling. Some of the materials in vaccines can cause temporary irritation. The actual vaccine material itself can cause your immune system to react with more *systemic*, or body-wide, symptoms. The following sections give you the basics on vaccine side effects.

REMEMBER

While certain side effects occur more commonly with some injections, just about any vaccine can cause a reaction. Contact your doctor or seek care in person if you have any concerns about side effects after a vaccine.

REMEMBER

Severe allergic reactions to vaccines are rare, occurring in about one person in a million. While being vigilant about a possible allergic reaction is sensible, remember that these types of reactions are quite rare. We discuss serious vaccine reactions later in this chapter.

Looking at common vaccine ingredients

Vaccines contain more than just what makes you immune to a particular disease. Any of these ingredients can cause some type of reaction. In general, the ingredients found in vaccines break down into five different categories:

>> **Antigens:** The substance that induces an immune response.

>> **Adjuvants:** Substances that tell your immune system to take notice of and respond to the antigen.

>> **Preservatives:** Substances that allow vaccines to remain stable and help prevent bacterial or fungal growth in multi-use vials.

>> **Stabilizers:** Substances that prevent the antigens from breaking down and becoming ineffective.

>> **Production materials:** These are used during the manufacturing of the vaccine but removed as much as possible before the vaccine is sent out. A vaccine may contain trace amounts of these materials.

All substances used in vaccines have been approved for use in the United States and deemed safe by the Food and Drug Administration (FDA).

Antigens and antigen reactions

Getting antigens into your body for your immune system to detect is the whole point of vaccinations. Our immune systems usually work silently without us even noticing. Many vaccine antigens do cause reactions we notice, sometimes serious ones. In general, vaccines that contain live but weakened bacteria or viruses are more likely to cause a reaction than those that contain killed viruses. Some live vaccines cause a very mild illness that is similar to the infection they are preventing.

Because antigens stimulate your immune system to make antibodies against a disease, they can cause systemic reactions such as fever or body aches.

Adjuvants

Adjuvants themselves don't do anything to make you immune to a disease. Instead, they are the flares and noisemakers that wake up your immune system to notice the antigens. This helps the antigens do their job more effectively by creating a stronger immune response.

One of the adjuvants commonly used is aluminum salts, used in over 20 different vaccines, including diphtheria, tetanus, and pertussis (DTaP), hepatitis B, and pneumococcal conjugate vaccines (see Chapter 6). These have been used for over 80 years. Vaccines containing aluminum may cause more temporary redness and hardness to the skin than other vaccines. (See the nearby sidebar "The aluminum and thimerosal additives" for more about aluminum in vaccines.)

Other adjuvants include oil-in-water emulsions and fat emulsions. Some vaccines use natural extracts. These include Chilean soapbark tree in the Shingrix shingles vaccine, and squalene from shark liver oil in a flu vaccine for the elderly (whose immune systems don't always make as strong an immune response otherwise).

These adjuvants are often designated only by letters and numbers rather than names, but they can be clearly identified. Examples include MF59 (squalene from shark liver oil), AS03 (also squalene), AS01B (Chilean soapbark tree mix), AS04 (fat and aluminum mix), and CpG 1018 (synthetic DNA that mimics genetic material from viruses or bacteria).

THE ALUMINUM AND THIMEROSAL ADDITIVES

The two vaccine ingredients that garner the most public attention include an adjuvant, aluminum, and a preservative, thimerosal:

- Aluminum salts have been used as an adjuvant in many vaccines for over seven decades. Aluminum is hardly an unusual substance; it's found in drinking water and many foods. In large quantities, aluminum can be *neurotoxic*, which means it can affect the brain. The average adult takes in 7 to 9 milligrams of aluminum a day from food and water.

  Children are the main focus of aluminum concerns. But studies show that in the first six months of life, a breastfed infant ingests 7 milligrams of aluminum, compared to 38 milligrams for formula-fed infants and almost 117 milligrams for infants on soy formula. By comparison, the total intake of aluminum from vaccines in the first six months of life equals just 4.4 milligrams. There's no scientific evidence that the aluminum in vaccines causes any harm.

- Thimerosal is a preservative that contains mercury, which can, in large amounts, also be neurotoxic. However, the form of mercury in thimerosal, ethylmercury, is less easily stored by the body, so it doesn't build up like methylmercury does. A vaccine containing 0.01 percent thimerosal contains about the same amount of mercury as is found in a can of tuna fish. Live vaccines don't contain any thimerosal.

  For twenty years, no vaccine has had thimerosal as an ingredient, except for the multi-use vials of the flu vaccine. The flu vaccine can be given from single-use vials without thimerosal. Unless a multi-use vial is used, no vaccine used in children has thimerosal as an ingredient.

  One maker of the adult and adolescent tetanus and diphtheria vaccine does use thimerosal in its manufacturing process to avoid bacterial growth, so trace amounts may appear in this particular manufacturer's vaccines.

  Thimerosal hasn't proven to be neurotoxic in any scientific studies. But manufacturers stopped using it; in fact, nearly all vaccines come in forms that are thimerosal free. No vaccine for infants under 6 months has thimerosal. All vaccines for children under 6 are available thimerosal free. Only the multi-use flu vaccine contains more than a trace amount of thimerosal, and single-use vaccines are available.

Preservatives

Like foods we keep on the shelves, sometimes preservatives are used so vaccines don't go bad and to keep bacteria from growing. These preservatives are used in very tiny amounts. Preservatives keep vaccines that come in multi-dose vials from becoming contaminated. Otherwise, just like milk left open in the fridge, vaccines can go bad, and bacteria can grow in the vials. A century ago, when vaccines were first being used, multi-use vials sometimes grew bacteria or fungi. Antibiotics are also sometimes used to keep vials, especially multi-use vials, from having bacterial growth.

Three preservatives are used in standard vaccines in the United States: phenol, 2-phenoxyethanol, and thimerosal.

>> **Phenol** is in a number of products commonly used — mouthwashes, throat lozenges, and throat sprays.

>> **2-phenoxyethanol** is used in some cosmetics and antiseptics and is used in only one polio vaccine.

>> **Thimerosal** contains mercury. It is used only in multi-use vials for the influenza vaccine. It is not used in any childhood vaccines, and there are thimerosal-free flu vaccines.

Mercury would be a concern if ingested in large amounts. There are two kinds of mercury: methylmercury and ethylmercury. Methylmercury can build up in your body and cause harm; ethylmercury, which is what is in thimerosal, is more easily excreted and less likely to cause harmful build-up. (See the nearby sidebar "The aluminum and thimerosal additives" for more details on thimerosal use in vaccines.)

Stabilizers

Stabilizers prevent what's in vaccines from breaking down as they travel from manufacturing sites around the world to your doctor's office. Vaccines can't be given right after they're produced. The logistics of packaging, shipping, and distributing a vaccine means it can be months or years before it's actually given. Changes in temperature and pH (measuring acidity and alkalinity) can destroy the active ingredients in vaccines without stabilizers.

Gelatin (like in Jell-O and other desserts) is a common stabilizer. It is likely the most common cause of vaccine allergic reactions, and those who are affected by it are likely to know that prior to getting vaccines. Other vaccines use sugars (lactose magnesium compounds and sorbitol). An allergy to any of these substances can potentially cause an allergic reaction, although the amounts used are small and such allergies are not common.

Production materials

Production materials include ingredients used in making the vaccine that are removed from the final product, leaving only trace amounts behind. Certain antibiotics, egg proteins, and formaldehyde are examples of production materials:

» **Antibiotics:** Antibiotics help prevent contamination during the manufacturing process. The antibiotics chosen to be in vaccines are not the ones that commonly cause allergies (like penicillin or sulfa drugs); instead, antibiotics like neomycin, polymyxin B, streptomycin, and gentamicin are used, which are not common causes of allergies, especially not when used in such minuscule amounts.

» **Egg proteins:** The oldest way to make a flu (or yellow fever) vaccine is to inject the virus into an egg to make copies of itself for use in making the antigens needed. This can result in a small amount of egg protein in these vaccines as well as in measles and mumps vaccines (such as the MMR, described in Chapter 6), which use eggs in production. In nearly all cases, you can still take these vaccines if you have an egg allergy, since very little egg remains in the vaccine. There are flu vaccines that do not use eggs — Flucelvax and Flublok — if you ever need an egg-free vaccine.

» **Formaldehyde:** Formaldehyde is used to inactivate toxins and viruses during the manufacturing process. A trace amount can be left in the vaccine, but it is less than we have naturally in our bodies.

REMEMBER

Always tell your doctor about any allergies. If you have concerns or a history of an allergy to a vaccine component, especially anaphylaxis, talk to your doctor. Your doctor may want to take further history and follow up with testing (like a scratch test with the vaccine or component if you had a serious allergic response) or have you be observed for 30 minutes after future vaccinations. For those with more serious allergies, especially those with anaphylaxis, it is best to wait in the doctor's office for 30 minutes after the injection. Reactions can occur even after this time period, but they're rare. A previous severe allergic reaction to a specific vaccine, like the flu vaccine, is a contraindication to receiving this vaccine again.

Distinguishing vaccine delivery methods

REMEMBER

Vaccines can be given in several different ways. Some vaccines have to be given by needles, but not all of them. Some have to be injected into the muscle, others just under the skin. Different needles are needed for different injections. If the wrong injection type is given, the vaccine may not be as effective.

You may experience different side effects, depending on the way the vaccine is administered. Here are the most common methods:

» **Intramuscular:** Most vaccines are given intramuscularly, or into a muscle. While this type of vaccination may cause the most initial pain, it can cause fewer local side effects like redness or swelling than vaccines given subcutaneously (into fat). Vaccines that are inactivated (not live) and vaccines that have adjuvants in them to increase the immune response are usually given in the muscle to avoid a skin reaction.

» **Intranasal:** A few vaccines, such as the live flu vaccine, are given in a nasal spray. While this may seem like a perfect vaccination method, intranasal vaccines can cause local reactions such as nasal congestion, cough, fever, headache, muscle aches, sore throat, vomiting, and wheezing.

» **Oral:** Some vaccines are given orally, in a liquid suspension. Oral vaccines can cause gastrointestinal symptoms such as nausea or vomiting. Some are an attenuated live vaccine, like typhoid or polio, which can create mild symptoms related to the gastrointestinal illness.

» **Subcutaneous:** These are injected into the fat rather than the muscle. The injections don't go as deep as intramuscular injections, but the subcutaneous area is more easily irritated.

» **Subdermal:** These injections go into the area just beneath the skin. Because the material is injected directly under the skin, a bubble, or *wheal,* can occur at the site, sometimes accompanied by local skin reactions such as redness or itching.

Watching for localized skin reactions

Reactions around the injection site are the most common types of vaccine reactions. While they're uncomfortable, they're rarely serious. Many people have pain, swelling, or redness. These reactions usually occur within hours of the injection and are usually mild; they don't require treatment. These reactions are not considered allergic reactions.

The following sections discuss localized skin reactions to vaccines in more detail.

Injection pain

Sometimes shots hurt. Injection pain can occur from the needlestick itself or from the medication as it's injected, stretching the muscle and causing inflammation. Some factors that can affect the pain from the needle itself include

>> **Whether the injection is intramuscular or subcutaneous:** To reach the muscle, the injector must use a larger needle. Subcutaneous injections don't go as deep and use a smaller needle. The adjuvants, which are usually only intramuscular, can cause more pain, making intramuscular shots more painful. (We cover vaccine delivery methods earlier in this chapter.)

>> **Whether the medication comes from a glass ampule or a vial with a rubber stopper:** A needle going through a rubber stopper can dull the needle point slightly. The sharper the needle, the less pain you feel.

>> **Whether it's warm or cold:** Cold medicines taken directly from the refrigerator can also cause more of a sting than material that's warmer.

>> **The site of the injection:** Small children are usually vaccinated on the thigh (and not on the buttock anymore) with a specific-sized needle. Older children and adults are vaccinated in the upper arm with a different-sized needle. Health professionals will know where to aim the shot in order to avoid any nerves. This is why we avoid the buttock to ensure the large sciatic nerve is not injured. Do report to your vaccinator if you feel what seems like nerve pain with the injection.

TIP

>> **Your own reaction:** Tightening up your muscles will make any injection hurt more. Distract yourself by looking the other way, singing the alphabet song, or anything else that takes your mind off the needle.

Itching

Itching can occur alone or in combination with redness and swelling at the injection site as a normal reaction to a foreign substance. It isn't usually a problem.

Hives

WARNING

Hives, raised bumps that come and go, can occur as a minor symptom after a vaccine or as part of a more serious systemic reaction. Some people — and you may already know it if you are one of them — are prone to developing hives. This is an allergic reaction (we cover such reactions later in this chapter).

Rash

If you discover a rash after a vaccine, it may be one of several things. Live vaccines, including those that cause a rash such as chicken pox or measles, are more likely to cause a rash, probably as a mild vaccine-induced case of the disease. Vaccines or ingredients that commonly cause rashes include the following:

>> **Antibiotics** found in some vaccines can also cause a generalized rash in those who have allergies. Neomycin, Polymyxin B, and streptomycin are used in some vaccines.

>> **Chicken pox vaccine** may cause a blister at the injection site in 3 percent of people or a more generalized rash in another 3 percent. This vaccine can also cause a delayed reaction, with rash and fever, that occurs one to four weeks or so after injection.

>> **MMR (measles, mumps, and rubella) vaccine** causes a short-term rash in about 5 percent of cases. Fever also happens in about one in ten children. Like the chicken pox vaccine, the MMR vaccine can cause a delayed reaction one to four weeks later with rash and fever.

>> **Tetanus and diphtheria toxoid vaccines** cause a rash or hives in 5 to 13 percent of recipients.

Rarely, vaccines for mumps/measles/rubella, diphtheria/pertussis/tetanus, hepatitis A and B, human papillomavirus, and meningitis cause a skin reaction called *erythema multiforme*. The lesions, which may resemble bull's-eyes and occur in patches, often don't cause any side effects, but they may itch or burn.

WARNING

In extremely rare cases, a serious skin reaction that causes a painful blistering over a large part of the body, which can include mucous membranes (eyes, mouth, nose, and/or genitals), is called Stevens-Johnson syndrome. If you have any type of rash besides a small, localized area of redness at the site after getting a vaccine, report it to your doctor.

Redness at the site

REMEMBER

When you have any type of insult to your skin, such as a cut, a bruise, or an injection, your body reacts with a typical inflammatory response that can cause redness. While this is usually a normal reaction, let your doctor know if the redness spreads, you run a fever, or you feel generally unwell.

WARNING

In rare cases, a vaccine may cause *cellulitis*, an infection of the skin itself at the injection site due to bacteria entering through the hole in your skin. If the area of redness enlarges or you're running a fever, call your doctor. If you are uncomfortable, an ice pack applied for 20 minutes at a time can help decrease your discomfort.

Swelling at the site

Several vaccines or the ingredients they're made of can cause swelling or lumps at the injection site. Vaccines containing aluminum hydroxide can cause small nodules under the skin if given subcutaneously that last up to a few months, which is why vaccines with adjuvants are usually given intramuscularly. A knot or lump at the injection site is generally not a concern if you have no other side effects. The DTaP vaccine, given to children in an arm or leg, can sometimes cause the entire limb to swell up.

Ice packs can be used to treat swelling at an injection site. Cover the ice bag so it isn't directly on the skin, and leave it on for no more than 20 minutes at a time.

Expecting a systemic immune response

Systemic responses can affect any part of your body. Vaccines often produce a systemic reaction as your immune system revs up making antibodies against the new invader. In the process, compounds that cause fever and other systemic side effects are released.

We refer to vaccines that cause this sort of reaction as *reactogenic.* These are the vaccines that create an immune reaction that we feel. The shingles vaccine, Shingrix, is known for being more reactogenic, as are some COVID-19 vaccines.

Although side effects are no fun to experience, think of them as a sign that your vaccination is working as it should to produce immunity. Common systemic effects include fever, headache, muscle aches, stomach issues, and tiredness, as you find out in the following sections.

There is a concern that taking fever and pain-reducing medications such as aspirin, ibuprofen, or acetaminophen before the injection can reduce your body's immune response. This may keep your immune system from responding to the vaccine and creating immunity. Taking anti-fever medications such as ibuprofen and acetaminophen *after* symptoms appear seems to allow the body's immune system time to work more effectively.

Checking for fever

Some vaccines may cause a transient rise in temperature. The diphtheria, tetanus, and pertussis vaccine (DTaP) can be associated with a fever in one in four children. A fever is a temperature above 100.4 degrees Fahrenheit. Fevers after vaccinations usually start within 24 hours and can last up to a few days. If you have a very high fever or feel generally unwell, report it to your doctor.

The fever can also be due to another illness, so do watch out for other symptoms unrelated to the vaccine.

It's okay for children to be vaccinated if they are feeling a little ill or have a low-grade fever; just talk to their healthcare provider first.

WARNING

Children can be given acetaminophen or ibuprofen for fever. Don't give aspirin; in rare instances, aspirin can increase the risk of a potentially serious condition called Reye's syndrome if given to children after vaccines, especially live vaccines such as varicella. Reye's syndrome can cause fever, irritability, fatigue, confusion, difficulty breathing, or seizures. Call 911 if your child has these symptoms.

REMEMBER

Make sure to stay hydrated if you have a fever. Children and the elderly in particular can become dehydrated quickly.

Having a headache

Vaccines often cause a temporary headache. Take acetaminophen or ibuprofen if your headache bothers you. Avoid aspirin, especially for children or adolescents, who may have had a live vaccine like varicella (chicken pox), MMR (measles, mumps, and rubella), or the live attenuated flu vaccine (nasal spray).

Waking up achy

Achy muscles often follow an injection as part of the systemic immune response. Mild painkillers such as acetaminophen or ibuprofen can help. In rare cases, the polio vaccine can cause temporary muscle weakness. Report any unusual weakness to your doctor.

Feeling fatigued

WARNING

Tiredness after a vaccine, like muscle achiness, is fairly common. Unusual fatigue, confusion, or losing consciousness is not. Report these immediately to your doctor as they can be a sign of a more serious complication.

Having gastrointestinal issues

WARNING

Gastrointestinal issues such as diarrhea, nausea, and vomiting can occur after some vaccines, especially oral vaccines. Intranasal vaccines can cause nasal congestion. Talk to your healthcare provider if symptoms last more than a day or two, or if you experience severe gastrointestinal symptoms. Report severe abdominal pain immediately, as this can be a sign of a potentially dangerous reaction.

Getting lightheaded or passing out

TIP

Some people are prone to passing out. If you're one of them, you may know this already. Anxiety about an injection and holding your breath can cause you to feel lightheaded or even faint. Pain from an injection or an allergic reaction can cause someone to pass out. Do sit down (or lie down) if you are feeling faint. Most who do faint (three in four) are adolescents. Fortunately, four in five who faint do so in the first 15 minutes after injection, so waiting in the doctor's office for 15 minutes after the vaccination can help prevent serious injuries from falling.

Recognizing and Treating Serious Reactions

Serious or possible life-threatening reactions rarely occur after vaccination, affecting one or two per million people. When they do, quick action can help. Knowing what to watch for can decrease your risk of serious harm. The following sections can help.

REPORTING VACCINE SIDE EFFECTS

The Vaccine Adverse Event Reporting System (VAERS), which started in 1990, tracks any adverse reactions from vaccines. Health professionals and manufacturers are required to report to VAERS any adverse reaction listed on the site, which has a Table of Reportable Event Following Vaccination. Individuals can also report reactions directly to the site. They're strongly encouraged to report any adverse event after vaccination, even if it's not clear whether the vaccine was responsible. Administration errors should also be reported.

Serious adverse reactions, according to the Food and Drug Administration (FDA), are reactions where "the patient outcome is death, life-threatening (real risk of dying), hospitalization (initial or prolonged), disability (significant, persistent, or permanent), congenital anomaly, or required intervention to prevent permanent impairment or damage."

Anyone can access information on the VAERS site: vaers.hhs.gov/index.html.

The National Vaccine Injury Compensation Program will also compensate patients and their families for specific side effects or injuries due to recommended vaccines. See www.hrsa.gov/vaccine-compensation/index.html for more information.

REMEMBER Reporting a reaction to your doctor, who will then report it to watchdog organizations such as the U.S. Food and Drug Administration (FDA) or other regulatory bodies in other countries, can reduce the risk of someone else having a similar reaction. See the nearby sidebar "Reporting vaccine side effects" for more info on how reporting agencies use information. You can report directly to these agencies as well, but talk to your doctor first in case you need medical treatment.

Avoiding allergic reactions

Allergic reactions can take many forms, from hives or rash to feeling short of breath, wheezing, abdominal pain, or facial swelling. Unfortunately, you may not know you have an allergy to one of the materials found in a vaccine until you actually receive a vaccine.

REMEMBER But in some cases, knowing you have an allergy and reporting it to your doctor can help prevent an allergic reaction. Vaccines can contain ingredients you may not expect them to, such as gelatin. If you know you have allergies, take the following precautions:

>> Make sure your doctor knows if you have allergies to any substance or if anyone else in your family has a reaction after receiving a vaccination.

>> If you have a history of severe allergies like anaphylaxis, always carry an epinephrine pen with you.

>> See whether your doctor wants you to wait in the clinic or pharmacy for 15–30 minutes after the vaccine, since most severe reactions occur shortly afterward.

WARNING Some vaccines have latex in the vial or syringe, which in rare cases can lead to an exposure that causes an allergic reaction. This includes some tetanus, meningitis, hepatitis A and B, and haemophilus influenzae type b (Hib) vaccines. The rotavirus oral droppers have latex as well. This may not be enough exposure to trigger an allergy in everyone allergic to latex, but it is worth discussing with your doctor if you have a severe latex allergy.

Anaphylactic reactions

Anaphylactic reactions can be deadly. While anaphylaxis is most likely to occur in someone with known allergies, an anaphylactic reaction can also occur in someone without such a history.

Anaphylactic reactions normally occur within a few minutes, usually within 15 minutes, after the vaccine. Symptoms include some of the same symptoms as an allergic reaction — hives, facial swelling, and difficulty breathing — but may escalate to include chest tightness, swelling of the throat and airway, trouble breathing, abdominal pain, nausea and vomiting, extremely low blood pressure, and passing out.

WARNING

Anaphylaxis is a true medical emergency. This is why for some vaccines you are asked to wait 15 to 30 minutes after receiving the vaccine so someone can respond immediately if you become ill. If you carry an epinephrine pen (EpiPen), administer it immediately. If you're still at the clinic or pharmacy, make someone aware of your symptoms at the first sign of a reaction. Those who are licensed to vaccinate are also trained in CPR to respond to a severe case of anaphylaxis. If you're not still at the doctor's office, call 911. Always call 911 after using an epinephrine pen.

Febrile seizures after childhood vaccinations

Febrile seizures are common in children. Between 2 and 5 percent of children have at least one before age 5, and this has nothing to do with vaccinations. About 40 percent of those who have one have more than one. These seizures can occur after anything that causes a fever. After vaccination, febrile seizures occur in about 1 in 30,000 children.

Vaccines more likely to cause fever are also more likely to cause a febrile seizure. For example, 1 in 3,000 children experience a febrile seizure after the measles vaccine, and fewer than 1 in 1,000 may have a febrile seizure after the DTaP vaccine.

REMEMBER

Febrile seizures can worry parents, but they don't generally cause long-term harm. If your child has a febrile seizure, you should do the following:

>> Place your child on the ground in a safe area and turn them on their side.

>> Don't try to restrain your child.

>> Don't place anything in their mouth. Trying to keep a child from biting their tongue isn't recommended.

>> Watch the time. If a seizure continues for more than five minutes, call 911.

>> If your child turns blue or isn't breathing, call 911.

>> After the seizure ends, notify your child's doctor. If this is your child's first febrile seizure, your child should be seen.

REMEMBER

Having a febrile seizure does not mean that your child has epilepsy. Most children who have febrile seizures do not go on to have epilepsy.

Guillain-Barré syndrome

Guillain-Barré syndrome, or GBS, affects nerve cells by causing your own immune system to attack them. It can cause muscle weakness and paralysis that are usually temporary but can require ventilation in an intensive care unit initially, and some residual damage may remain. It often occurs after a viral illness.

There was an increase of cases of GBS after swine flu vaccination in 1976, to about 1 in 100,000. Since 1976, GBS has not been a worry. At most, one or two in a million who are vaccinated for the flu may develop GBS, but having the influenza infection itself is likely a greater risk. GBS often occurs after a viral illness, including after influenza, but particularly after a gastrointestinal infection called *Campylobacter jejuni*. Adults over age 50 have the highest chance of developing GBS.

REMEMBER

GBS can develop days or weeks after a vaccine. Report any new weakness to your doctor. If you're having trouble breathing, call 911. If you have had GBS before, please talk to your doctor before being vaccinated.

SIDS AND VACCINES: NO CONNECTION EXISTS

Every year, babies between the ages of 2 and 4 months die of Sudden Infant Death Syndrome, or SIDS. This is also the age where many babies receive multiple vaccinations, leading some people to question whether there is a connection.

No connection between SIDS and vaccine timing has ever been found. The best ways to protect your baby against SIDS are as follows:

- Place your baby on his back to sleep.
- Keep pillows, blankets, soft crib toys, and crib bumper out of your baby's crib.
- Don't sleep with your baby in your bed.
- Use a firm mattress for your baby's crib.

Thrombocytopenia

Thrombocytopenia is a decrease in the platelet count and can be caused by an autoimmune reaction. Platelets are small blood fragments that assist in blood clotting. There is an increased risk of thrombocytopenia in children who receive the MMR vaccine, although the risk is low, occurring in the six weeks following an MMR vaccination in about one in 40,000 vaccinated.

Symptoms can include

>> Increased or unexplained bleeding or bruising

>> A rash made up of reddish pinpoint dots or purplish patches

>> Blood in urine or stools

>> Bleeding from gums or nose (including with brushing your teeth)

REMEMBER

Report symptoms to your child's doctor immediately.

Looking at Multiple Vaccines and the Immune System

Infancy used to come with a lot more risks. Parents knew surviving infancy was far from a given. We now have a lot more protections against these infectious diseases thanks to vaccines.

The protections for infants from vaccines have increased. Half a century ago, babies received five vaccinations — diphtheria, pertussis, tetanus, polio, and smallpox — and around eight vaccine injections by their second birthday. Today, babies are protected against 14 diseases, with over 20 vaccine injections by age 2.

The 14 diseases infants are protected against include measles, mumps, rubella, rotavirus, varicella (chicken pox), tetanus, pertussis (whooping cough), hepatitis A, hepatitis B, haemophilus influenzae type b(Hib), diphtheria, pneumococcus, polio, and influenza. Some of these used to take many infant lives but now are much less common thanks to vaccines. (Flip to Chapter 8 for more about vaccines for children.)

With more protection comes more vaccines. Infants receive more vaccines in their first year of life than before. Infants are given multiple vaccines at the same time, at young ages. Numerous studies have looked to see whether multiple vaccines given on the same day, or combined together, like the MMRV vaccine, overwhelm or cause any type of damage to a child's immune system. The studies have shown they do not.

Babies start to develop their immune systems in the womb. Types of cells that trigger an immune reaction are found as early as the 14th week of pregnancy. Infants begin to initiate immune responses very quickly after birth; babies given hepatitis B vaccines right at birth generate a very strong immune response.

REMEMBER

Can you overwhelm a baby's immune system by giving it too many types of vaccines at once? Studies say no. Vaccinated children are not more likely than unvaccinated children to develop infections they are not vaccinated against.

An average baby — if there were such a thing — is actually exposed to fewer antigens via vaccine than babies were even 40 years ago. We use a lot fewer antigens in each vaccine. Thirty years ago, vaccines used 3,000 antigens to protect against those eight diseases by age 2. Today vaccines use about one-tenth that number to protect against 14 diseases by age 2.

This is thanks to the eradication of smallpox and the advancement of chemistry, which allow us to use just the most important bacterial or viral parts and not the whole (living or killed) bacterium or virus itself.

REMEMBER

Infants are also not challenged by the many natural infections that used to be so dangerous for them and led to so many infant deaths. If your child has an immune deficiency disorder or is sick, talk to your doctor about his vaccine scheduling.

3

Scheduling Safety

IN THIS PART . . .

Recognize the importance of childhood vaccines.

Keep current with adult vaccines.

Know when to avoid vaccines.

Debunk a variety of vaccine myths.

Chapter **8**

Vaccines for Children

C hildhood comes with lots of milestones. Children grow bigger and stronger each day. Vaccines are part of growing up safely and are milestones in development. In this chapter, we give you the facts to understand current guidelines for childhood vaccines. We also discuss the immunity your baby gets from you against certain diseases, and how long these immunities generally last.

Understanding Mom-to-Baby Immunity

Babies come into the world with some immunity, called *passive immunity*, for specific infections from their mothers. Antibodies that mom has from vaccines or from getting sick herself can be found in her baby at birth. Unfortunately, these antibodies don't last forever, and some are all gone by 3 months. Passive immunity lasts at most a few months, although breastfeeding can increase how long a baby is protected. Also unfortunately, only certain antibodies cross the placenta to reach the baby from mom. IgM antibodies from very recent infections are too big to cross the placenta. (*IgM* stands for immunoglobulin M; these are the first antibodies produced in response to a new infection or a vaccine.)

Breastfeeding benefits

Breastfeeding your baby, even for a short time, can help them develop immunity to diseases. That said, breastfed is always best, and colostrum, the yellowish first fluid produced by a mom after birth, is especially rich in antibodies. And the longer you breastfeed, the more antibodies your baby gets, because antibodies continue to pass through the breast milk as long as you're nursing.

In addition, breastfed babies seem to develop stronger immune responses, which increases their immunity to a disease after a vaccine. Breastfed babies also mount a stronger immune response to common childhood illnesses.

Antibodies passed on during pregnancy

If you've had certain diseases, or been immunized against them, you will pass a temporary passive immunity to your baby during the last three months of pregnancy. This immunity will last for a while, but without doing bloodwork, knowing just how long it lasts is impossible. Certainly don't assume your baby is protected against any of these dangerous diseases:

>> Chicken pox

>> Influenza

>> Measles

>> Mumps

>> Pertussis

>> Rubella

>> Tetanus

In some cases, passive immunity wears off very quickly, within a few weeks. This is why immunizations against pertussis (whooping cough) and Hib begin at 2 months. (*Hib* is the easier way to say Haemophilus influenzae type b.) If your baby has maternal antibodies to diseases that convey longer immunity, such as measles or chicken pox, the antibodies your baby carries can make the vaccine ineffective.

The current United States vaccination schedule has been created taking all these factors into account, which is why it's important that you follow the schedule correctly. Keep reading to find out more about U.S. vaccination schedules.

Getting a Reminder of the Effectiveness and Importance of Vaccinations

Babies come into the world fragile, and we feel the need to protect and cocoon them. Parents want to do everything they can to shield their children from dangers. One of the first ways we are able to protect fragile babies is through vaccination on the first day of life.

Most parents today have never had to experience many terrible illnesses because vaccines have worked. Rest assured that every injection given is given for a good reason. Numerous studies have made sure that the vaccine schedules today are safe, even with multiple jabs on the same day.

Your baby actually receives fewer *antigens* — the active parts of vaccines that cause your baby to become immune to certain diseases — than babies who were vaccinated 50 years ago. Through science, we have been better able to target vaccines and use fewer antigens.

WARNING

Most vaccines can cause mild side effects, such as soreness or redness at the injection site, a mild fever, muscle aches, tiredness, and crankiness in young children. More serious reactions should always be reported immediately to your child's health provider. See Chapter 7 for more information.

REMEMBER

Ear infections, mild cold symptoms, and other mild illnesses usually aren't a contradiction to giving a vaccine. Before any vaccination, tell your doctor if your child has an allergic reaction to any substance in the vaccine (or if allergies to certain substances run in your family).

REMEMBER

It may not seem like the first priority to vaccinate your new baby against diseases you've never even seen in your lifetime. This is especially true if there's any concern about side effects. But in all cases, the risk of not vaccinating your child outweighs the risk of forgoing vaccines. (See Chapter 11 for more about the myths related to vaccination risks.) More detail on each of the vaccines in this chapter can be found in Chapter 6.

Focusing on Vaccinations in the First Year of Life

On your baby's first visit to her health provider, you may receive a small booklet to record all her vaccinations in. While your doctor will also keep a vaccination record, it's important that you keep this little booklet up to date as well. If you have to move, your doctor suddenly decides to retire, or you want to switch doctors, it's good to have this information at your fingertips.

It's also handy to have as your child ages. Your child's schools may want to make sure her vaccinations are up to date. Your teen may call from his summer job two states away wanting to know when his last tetanus shot was, because he's at the emergency department and the doctor needs to know now. Many adults still use their childhood vaccine cards.

TECHNICAL STUFF

Recording this information in your child's baby book is also fine, but as a mother of five, I (coauthor Sharon) can almost guarantee that you'll stop adding vaccination information by the time your baby goes to kindergarten. Sooner if they're not your first baby, of course. If they're your fifth, it's unlikely that anything beyond their name will ever make it into a baby book.

In this section, we discuss the first-year vaccination schedule and how it came to be. Table 8-1 shows the first-year vaccination schedule at a glance.

TABLE 8-1

First-Year Vaccination Schedule at a Glance

Vaccination	Age Given
Hepatitis B	Birth, 1–2 months, and 6–18 months
Rotavirus	2, 4, and maybe* 6 months
DTaP	2, 4, and 6 months
Hib	2, 4, maybe* 6, and 12–15 months
Inactivated polio virus (IPV)	2, 4, and 6–18 months
Influenza	6 months or older (2 doses 4 weeks apart, then yearly)
Pneumococcal conjugate (PCV13)	2, 4, 6, and 12–15 months

(depending on vaccine used)

Hepatitis B

We have had vaccines for hepatitis B only since the 1980s. The disease can cause permanent and serious liver damage. A blood- and other bodily fluid-borne disease, hepatitis B infects as many as 2 million people in the United States, or one of 172 people. Many don't even know they have the disease. Hepatitis B can cause serious liver damage, and children under age 5 who develop this disease have a 15 percent to 25 percent chance of prematurely dying from it. A hepatitis B positive mom can transmit the infection to her baby during childbirth.

The first vaccine against hepatitis B is given within the first 24 hours of life. The second dose is given at 1 to 2 months, and the third between 6 and 18 months. Three injections are 95 percent effective in preventing hepatitis B for your child's lifetime. In most cases, this vaccine causes only mild side effects.

The timing of the vaccine can vary, depending on mom's hepatitis B status and the baby's birthweight:

>> All healthy newborns whose moms are hepatitis B negative and who weigh over 2,000 grams (approximately 4 pounds, 6 ounces) should receive this vaccine within 24 hours after birth.

>> If mom's hepatitis status is unknown, the vaccine should be given within 12 hours after birth.

>> If mom has hepatitis B, the newborn should receive the vaccine within 24 hours, regardless of birthweight.

WARNING

Premature babies under 2,000 grams or sick newborns whose moms are hepatitis B negative should be given the vaccine at 1 month or before they're discharged from the hospital.

Rotavirus

Rotavirus causes a gastrointestinal infection that can be serious in young children, causing fever, diarrhea, and vomiting. It's especially dangerous in infants because they can become dehydrated so easily. Before 2006, when the vaccine was introduced, rotavirus resulted in as many as 70,000 hospitalizations a year in the United States. Nearly all children had at least one bout with rotavirus before age 5.

Rotavirus is extremely contagious and easily passed via the oral-fecal route. Rotavirus can easily spread among small children, especially those in diapers. Because of the dangers of vomiting and diarrhea in infants, rotavirus vaccinations are started early at age 2 months. Your baby needs two or three doses of the vaccine, depending on the manufacturer. The three-dose variety covers multiple strains (G1, G2, G3, G4, and G9), and the two-dose variety covers just the most common strain (G1).

The rotavirus vaccine is easier to give than others. It comes as just drops in the mouth. (See Chapter 7 for more on oral vaccines.) This vaccine can be given at the same time as other vaccinations, such as the hepatitis B, Hib, pneumococcal conjugate, and polio vaccines.

Whereas many children used to be hospitalized with rotavirus each year, now nine in ten are protected from severe rotavirus (fever, vomiting, severe diarrhea, dehydration), and seven to eight out of ten are completely protected from the illness.

After having the vaccine, which is a live vaccine, some children may have mild diarrhea. The vaccine has also been associated with something called *intussusception*, which means one part of the bowel slides inside the other, like a telescope, causing a blockage. The rate of intussusception has not changed in infants since the vaccine was first introduced, but there is a tiny risk with vaccination that it may occur about a week after the vaccine is given. This is rare; intussusception in the week after vaccination may occur in between one in 20,000 to one in 100,000 infants in the United States. This can cause permanent bowel damage and requires immediate medical attention. The condition can usually be corrected by a doctor pushing air or fluid into the intestine (an enema guided by imaging) or in some cases by surgery.

WARNING

If a child has developed intussusception, they may show signs of stomach pain with severe crying. Some babies may pull their legs up to their chest. There may even be a lump in the abdomen. These episodes may come and go, even multiple times in the same hour, as the intestine may slide back and forth. There may be blood in the stool (but not always), which can be referred to as "red currant jelly" because of the blood and mucus in it. It's important to seek medical attention right away for these symptoms.

REMEMBER

All healthy infants starting at age 2 months should get this vaccine. It should be finished up by 8 months. Babies can have the vaccine if they have a mild cold or other mild illness. Babies who are moderately ill, especially with diarrhea or vomiting, should wait until they have gotten better.

WARNING

Who shouldn't get this vaccine?

>> Babies who have had a previous allergic reaction to the vaccine

>> Babies with documented allergies to any ingredients in the vaccine

>> Babies who have had a previous episode of intussusception

>> Babies who have severe combined immunodeficiency (SCID)

Talk to your doctor if your child has cancer, takes medications that affect the immune system, or has HIV/AIDS or another immune system issue. It may be fine to take the vaccine, but it's best to check.

DTaP (Diphtheria, tetanus, pertussis)

DTaP stands for diphtheria, tetanus, and pertussis (whooping cough). This is one of those vaccines that it seems like your child needs every time you go to the doctor, because children need five doses before age 6 to be safe from these diseases. DTaP vaccines are given at 2, 4, and 6 months in the first year, between 15 and 18 months, and then again between ages 4 and 6.

Diphtheria, tetanus, and pertussis are all serious diseases with a high death or disability rate:

>> **Diphtheria** can cause a child to choke and not be able to breathe. The death rate is between 5 percent and 10 percent. In the 1920s, between 13,000 and 15,000 people died each year from diphtheria.

>> **Tetanus** develops if a wound becomes infected with *Clostridium tetanus,* a bacterium. Tetanus can cause paralysis or extreme convulsions. Babies born to mothers who haven't been vaccinated against tetanus can develop neonatal tetanus if the umbilical stump becomes infected. Neonatal tetanus mortality is around 100 percent without medical care, even 50 percent worldwide with hospital care. Around 11 percent of people infected with tetanus die.

>> **Pertussis,** or whooping cough, can make babies stop breathing. There may be no cough when a baby gets sick. For older children, it can cause a cough that makes breathing, eating, or drinking very difficult. Between 2008 and 2011, around 3,000 infants developed pertussis each year, and around 16 died, most under the age of 3 months.

In addition to the typical vaccine injection reactions, the DTaP vaccines can cause some potentially concerning reactions. Uncontrollable crying for several hours, a high fever, or swelling of the arm or leg where the vaccination was given may occur.

WARNING

In extremely rare cases, seizures can occur after this vaccine. Always report any change in your child's level of consciousness or any possible seizure activity to your doctor immediately.

All children up to age 7 should be given this vaccine series. Babies with minor illnesses at the time can be given the vaccine.

WARNING

Contraindications to the DTaP vaccine include the following:

>> Any severe allergic reaction to the vaccine or a component of the vaccine previously

> » Previously went into a coma or had decreased consciousness or prolonged seizures within one week of receiving the vaccine, without another cause identified

REMEMBER

Do talk to your doctor if your child currently has a moderate or severe illness, has developed any sort of paralysis or severe allergic reaction after a prior dose, has uncontrolled seizures, or a deteriorating neurologic condition. These are rare, but it's important to discuss these before vaccination if they apply.

Hib

The Hib vaccine protects against bacterial infections that can make young children quite ill. Some kids have only mild symptoms, such as bronchitis or ear infections. However, the bacterium was the leading cause of meningitis in children under age 5 before the vaccine. Hib can also cause a life-threatening swelling of the epiglottis (the flap of tissue at the back of the throat), making children struggle to breathe. It can cause severe pneumonia, blood infections, and other severe illnesses.

Healthcare providers give the vaccine in a series of three or four injections, depending on the brand, starting at age 2 months and usually finishing the series at 12–15 months. Kids over age 5 don't usually get the vaccine unless they have health issues such as sickle cell anemia, HIV, or a history of a bone marrow transplant.

IPV (inactivated polio vaccine)

IPV, the polio vaccine, is another vaccination that your baby seems to need every time you turn around. This vaccine is given at 2 and 4 months, then again between 6 and 18 months, and at 4 to 6 years.

This vaccine is called IPV because it differs from the oral polio vaccine, called the Sabin vaccine, which was made from live material. IPV is the only polio vaccine used in the United States since 2000. The oral polio live vaccine is still used in some other parts of the world.

TECHNICAL STUFF

Most parents today have no memory of polio, but your parents may, and your grandparents certainly do. President Franklin D. Roosevelt was paralyzed from it. Polio cases usually occurred in the summer; in the summer of 1955, one hospital, Boston Children's Hospital, admitted over 650 children for polio.

The only reason to delay or not give the IPV is a previous allergic reaction to any of the ingredients. Mildly ill babies can receive the vaccine.

THE SHOT-TO-SUGAR-TO-SHOT HISTORY OF THE POLIO VACCINES

As a child, you may have received your polio vaccine on a sugar cube. Today, your child gets theirs as a shot, just like their grandmother did. Are we going backward? No, the polio protection story is an interesting one that has played out within most of our lifetimes. Good reasons exist for the back-and-forth changes in vaccination methods.

Polio was a terrifying disease that most often affected children. In 1952, over 58,000 cases were reported in the United States, with 3,200 dying and 21,000 left with permanent damage. Demand for a vaccine was high.

Jonas Salk created the first polio vaccine, which, like the current polio vaccine, was made from inactivated material. I (coauthor Sharon) vividly remember standing in line outside the firehouse with every other child in town to receive the first vaccine. Five million children were vaccinated by July 1955.

As much of a breakthrough as the first vaccine was, there were concerns that it wouldn't last long against the three common forms of poliovirus. A live vaccine created by Albert Sabin was deemed to last longer, necessitating fewer boosters, and to act more rapidly. There was even the thought that, since the live vaccine passed through stool, it might provide passive immunity to people in undeveloped countries through sewage.

By the 1960s there was some concern that the Sabin vaccine caused a small number of adults receiving the vaccine to develop cases of vaccine-induced polio. The debate over the best method to use and the refining of the Salk vaccine, which used monkey kidney cells from live monkeys to produce a more potent vaccine, went on for decades.

By 2000, the United States switched back to the Salk vaccine, now produced by using previously created monkey cell lines. At this point, it seems that the IPV has taken the race, and that polio as a disease will soon be completely eradicated. Just 22 cases were reported worldwide in 2017, thanks to global vaccination programs, but this number jumped in 2019 and 2020 to over 100 cases a year.

Influenza

The influenza vaccine needs to be given every year because the viruses causing the flu change from year to year. Since kids under age 2 have a high risk of complications from having the flu, it's important to start your baby's flu vaccine yearly once they reach the age of 6 months. When getting the vaccine for the first time, they'll need a follow-up injection four weeks after the first.

Symptoms of flu in babies may differ somewhat from those of adults. While babies may still run a fever, be irritable and achy, and have a cough or sore throat, they're more likely than adults to have vomiting and diarrhea as well.

Having your baby vaccinated against influenza is especially important if they're at high risk because of other health issues. These can include the following:

>> Asthma or other chronic lung disease

>> Heart disease

>> Immune system deficiencies

>> Kidney disorders

>> Liver disorders

>> Metabolic disorders

>> Neurological or neurodevelopmental issues, such as cerebral palsy

>> Obesity

REMEMBER

Complications of flu can be life-threatening in infants. Your baby can become dehydrated, run a very high fever, develop pneumonia, or have seizures. It takes about two weeks for the flu vaccine to protect your baby, so get the vaccine before flu season starts.

PCV13

The PCV13 vaccine (short for pneumococcal conjugate) protects against 13 types of pneumococcal bacteria. These 13 bacteria cause the most common types of pneumonia, which can cause serious respiratory illness in infants and children under age 2. The vaccine series consists of four injections, starting at age 2 months and finishing at 12–15 months.

Ask your doctor whether your baby should get the vaccine during an illness. A simple cold or other mild illnesses don't usually prevent your baby from getting the vaccine. Kids who've experienced a severe allergic reaction from a previous PCV13 vaccine shouldn't take the vaccine. Typical side effects include redness or soreness at the injection site or a mild fever.

Knowing New Vaccinations for Toddlers

Toddlerhood — the period from age 12 months to around 3 years — brings many changes. But one thing that doesn't change is your child's need for more vaccinations. Some vaccines are booster doses of vaccines started in the first year of life;

others are given for the first time once your child reaches 12 months. Repeat vaccines include

>> Hepatitis B, given at 12–18 months, if all three injections haven't already been completed

>> DTaP, given at 15–18 months

>> Hib, given at 12–15 months

>> IPV, third dose given at 6–18 months

>> Influenza, given yearly

>> PCV13, given at 12–15 months

By this age, toddlers may also have discovered that the healthcare provider's office isn't always a fun place, and now that they're mobile and more suspicious, you may actually have to hold them down for injections, adding insult to injury for them and temporary guilt for you.

TIP

Following are a few things you can do to help your toddler — and you — make it through injections with fewer tears and fears:

>> **Hold your toddler during the injection.** Once toddlers turn into wailing, writhing octopuses with numerous flailing limbs, this may not be possible. Hold them firmly but not too tightly. Standing them between your legs, facing you, may work once they're steady on their feet, as long as they don't dissolve into a mass of jelly when you try this.

>> **Use distraction.** If your toddler is still taking a bottle or breastfeeding, these can serve as distractors. Blowing bubbles, reading a book, bringing out a new toy, or having someone else make silly faces can be distracting.

>> **Bring their lovey.** By this age, many toddlers have a favorite object — a ratty corner of blanket, a falling-apart stuffed animal, or a piece of clothing they're attached to. Have it at the ready to give them the moment the injection is over. Are you beginning to get the feeling that you need to be an octopus yourself? You're right; parenthood is all about multitasking!

>> **Put a cool cloth over the injection site.** Never put ice directly on your child's skin without wrapping it in cloth first, and keep it on no longer than 20 minutes at a time. As your child gets a bit older, a bandage with a superhero on it may turn tears into smiles.

>> **Consider bribery.** Offer a cookie, a sucker, or some other rare treat after the injection. A little sugar can help reduce the sting, in your child's mind, at least.

>> **Give a pain reliever.** Giving ibuprofen or acetaminophen after the injection may be helpful if your child has a mild fever or other symptoms. Giving it beforehand can reduce the effectiveness of the vaccine.

Table 8-2 gives you an overview of the toddler vaccination schedule. Many of these vaccines are covered earlier in this chapter; this section covers the rest.

TABLE 8-2   ## Toddler Vaccination Schedule at a Glance

Vaccination	Age Given
MMR	12–15 months
Varicella	12–15 months
Hepatitis A	12–15 months, second dose six months later
Hepatitis B	12–18 months, third dose, if not already given
Hib	12–15 months
Influenza	Every year
IPV	6-18 months (third dose)
DTaP	15–18 months (fourth dose)
PCV13	12–15 months (third dose)

MMR (measles, mumps, rubella)

The MMR (or measles, mumps, rubella) vaccination is an important part of a toddler's vaccine schedule. This vaccine is given between the ages of 12 and 15 months; another booster is given to school-age and high school children.

The MMR vaccine can be given as the MMRV vaccine, which includes the vaccine against varicella, or chicken pox. (See the next section for details.) The most common symptoms of the MMR vaccine are similar to those of most vaccines, and include

>> Fever

>> Irritability

>> Redness or itching at the injection site

>> Soreness at the injection site

Reactions specific to each disease are listed in the following sections. A single dose of this vaccine is 93 percent effective against measles, 78 percent effective against mumps, and 97 percent effective against rubella. Receiving two shots increases immunity against measles to 97 percent and mumps to 88 percent.

Measles

The MMR vaccine isn't usually given before 12 months because your baby's immune system will be more receptive at one year.

There is one exception to this, however. If there's a measles outbreak in your area or you are traveling, your baby can be given an extra dose of the vaccine as early as 6 months, and then repeated at 12 months. The early dose isn't counted as one of the vaccines given on the vaccination schedule.

Measles is extremely contagious; 90 percent of people who come in contact with someone with measles will catch it. Measles also spreads easily through the air, so you can catch it from someone with whom you've had no direct contact.

Symptoms of measles include a high fever, a rash, watery red eyes, and a cough, and can last over a week. In rare cases, measles can cause brain infection (*encephalitis*), severe ear infection, pneumonia, or even death.

WARNING

The measles part of this vaccine can cause some potentially serious side effects, although these are rare. They include possible febrile seizures, which happen in one out of 3,000 cases, and a drop in platelet count, which occurs in one out of 30,000 cases. (These are addressed in more detail in Chapter 6.)

The vaccine can also lead to a fever in 10 percent and a rash in 5 percent of children. Your child can still go to day care or school with the rash. It can't spread.

Mumps

Many jokes have been made about the swollen "chipmunk cheeks" of a mumps sufferer, but the truth isn't at all funny. The facial swelling, which affects between 31 percent and 65 percent of people with mumps, is painful, and mumps can cause, in addition to fever, achiness and headache, permanent hearing loss, encephalitis, and swelling in the testes or ovaries. This infection can cause a reduction in fertility in boys when they become men and want to have their own families. Before the mumps vaccine, the disease also caused around 20 percent of all cases of viral meningitis in the United States. Rarely, mumps can lead to death.

Like the measles vaccine, the mumps vaccine is also a live one. Live vaccines can cause mild symptoms similar to the disease, including minor swelling in the cheeks. Side effects such as these usually show up around two weeks after vaccination and are uncommon.

Rubella

Rubella (German measles) and rubeola (regular measles) are sometimes confused, although their symptoms are quite different. Unlike measles, rubella is generally a mild disease, with a rash that begins on the face and spreads downward, a low-grade fever, possible pink eye, and a sore throat.

WARNING

But the major concern with rubella is its potential effect on pregnant women. Rubella can cause miscarriage or serious birth defects in an unborn baby whose mom has rubella. Pregnant women should absolutely not get the rubella vaccine. If you get the vaccine, it's imperative that you do not get pregnant for a month or more afterward. The rubella vaccine is a live vaccine and can cause a mild case of rubella, harming the unborn baby. (See Chapter 9 for adult vaccine requirements and risks.)

Before the rubella vaccine became available, in 1964–1965, 12.5 million people contracted rubella in a single year. It caused birth defects and also deafness in children born from mothers infected. Like regular measles, rubella is extremely contagious.

Rubella has now been eliminated in the Americas thanks to vaccination. The virus continues to spread elsewhere, especially as rubella has only been newly added to many vaccine programs around the world.

Who shouldn't get the MMR vaccine as a toddler

WARNING

Because the MMR is a combination vaccine, there are more contraindications to its use. Toddlers should not get the vaccine unless their healthcare provider gives the green light if they

>> Had a previous severe allergic reaction to any part of the vaccine

>> Have a severely compromised immune system, but persons with HIV and not AIDS can be vaccinated

There may be other reasons a healthcare provider may delay vaccination for a toddler, including if they

>> Had a blood transfusion within the last three months

>> Have very low platelets (which help our blood clot)

>> Need immediate testing for latent tuberculosis

>> Have received another live vaccine within the last four weeks

>> Are moderately ill — the doctor can make the call on whether or not to wait

Varicella or MMRV

The varicella, or chicken pox, vaccine can be given in combination with the MMR vaccine (see the previous section) or as a separate injection. Like the MMR vaccine, varicella is a live vaccine and is given at age 12–15 months because moms who have had the disease or been vaccinated provide some immunity to their babies. Kids get a booster at 4–6 years old.

Some parents feel that chicken pox is such a mild disease that just letting your child catch it is the best policy. And while it's true that chicken pox is usually a mild, although annoying, disease, in some cases, it can have serious complications, especially in infants and elderly adults who get it but also in children who have developed other medical issues. And the chicken pox vaccine can prevent adults from developing shingles later in life.

One difficult thing to watch as a doctor is a parent watching their child in an intensive care unit, trying to say they thought they were helping their child by not vaccinating for chicken pox. They didn't know their child would, as an adolescent, develop an autoimmune disorder or leukemia. They didn't know it could end up this bad.

Before the chicken pox vaccine became available, around 2 million people caught chicken pox each year, around 11,000 people were hospitalized with the disease, and between 100 and 150 died.

Side effects of the varicella vaccine, outside of the typical reactions such as fever and soreness, can include a rash around the site of the vaccine.

WARNING

Don't give your baby any products containing aspirin after this vaccine. Use acetaminophen or ibuprofen for mild side effects. Aspirin products can, in some cases, cause a rare and serious complication called Reye's syndrome.

Every healthy toddler should get the chicken pox vaccine at age 12 to 15 months.

WARNING

There are a few possible contraindications to the varicella vaccine for your toddler. They include

>> Toddlers who have had a severe allergic reaction to a component of the vaccine

>> Toddlers who have compromised immune systems

>> Toddlers who are currently ill or have a fever

>> Toddlers with untreated active tuberculosis

>> Toddlers who have had other live vaccines within the past four weeks

Talk to your doctor about vaccinating for varicella if you have any doubts about giving the vaccine to your toddler.

Hepatitis A

You may not think of hepatitis A as a disease that affects babies, but even in the United States, where a vaccine is available, up to 17,500 people, many of them children, become ill with this disease each year. Your toddler can be infected with hepatitis A by eating or drinking something contaminated with it, or via the fecal-oral route from another person. Childcare centers or nursery schools are common places for hepatitis A to spread.

Hepatitis A affects the liver; adults are more likely to show symptoms than children. Hepatitis A can last as long as six months, causing fever, diarrhea, vomiting, lack of appetite, yellowing of the whites of the eyes, fatigue, or joint pain.

Two injections, six months apart, are necessary for your toddler to develop full immunity to hepatitis A. If you're traveling with your baby to an area where hepatitis A is very common, your doctor may recommend giving the vaccine as early as age 6 months.

All children age 12 to 15 months should receive this vaccine. Side effects, outside of the typical sore arm and mild fever, are rare.

WARNING

Toddlers who have had a severe allergic reaction to any of the ingredients in the vaccine should not get it.

Surveying a Few Vaccines for Ages 4 to 6

Kids between the ages of 4 and 6 still need vaccines, although fortunately, they need fewer than they did as infants and toddlers. No new vaccines are introduced in this age group. See Table 8-3 for an overview.

TIP

Some schools require that your child be up to date on vaccines before attending. Each state has its own rules about vaccination. Because the laws can change, it's best to check your own state's website for information about their policies. The Immunization Action Coalition has data on all the state's requirements at www. immunize.org/laws/.

TABLE 8-3

Vaccines Given Between Ages Four and Six

Vaccination	Dose
DTaP	Fifth dose
IPV	Fourth dose
Influenza	Given yearly; children receiving their first dose will need two, four weeks apart
MMR	Second dose
Varicella	Second dose

Many states have opt-out laws for parents who don't want to immunize or who don't want to have their child have certain vaccines. An up-to-date list can be found at the National Conference of State Legislatures site at www.ncsl.org/research/health/school-immunization-exemption-state-laws.aspx.

Adding Some School-Age Vaccinations

The need for vaccinations drops off sharply for school-age kids. The only vaccine given regularly in the 7–10 age group is the flu vaccine. At 11–12, there's an increase in vaccinations, including two new vaccines and one booster that's slightly different from its predecessors. Check out Table 8-4 for an overview.

TABLE 8-4

Vaccines at a Glance from Age 7 to 12

Vaccination	Age Given
Influenza	Every year
Human papillomavirus	Age 11 to 12
Meningococcal conjugate (MenACWY)	Age 11 to 12
Tetanus, diphtheria, and pertussis (Tdap)	Age 11 to 12

Human papillomavirus (HPV)

As much as parents often dread thinking about it, the next few years are when many children become sexually active. One very common sexually transmitted disease that can affect both boys and girls is human papillomavirus (HPV), which causes genital warts. In 2018, there were 48 million diagnosed cases of HPV, many in older teens and people in their early 20s. HPV is so common that it will affect nearly every sexually active person at some point without the vaccine.

HPV can cause cervical, vaginal, vulvar, and anal cancer in women and penile and anal cancer in men. Both sexes can also develop throat or tonsil cancer from oral sex.

The HPV vaccine is generally started at 11 or 12, but can be given as early as age 9. A second dose is given any time more than six months after the first dose. The vaccine has no side effects outside of the usual soreness at the injection site.

Meningococcal conjugate (MenACWY)

A vaccine that helps protect against a type of bacterial meningitis caused by bacteria called *Neisseria meningitidis* is first given at age 11 to 12. Meningococcal bacteria can live harmlessly in up to 10 percent of people's nose and throat. But the bacteria can spread to the brain, spinal column, or blood, causing a serious illness that is rapidly fatal in 10 percent to 15 percent of patients, and leaving up to 20 percent of survivors with long-term damage. (See Chapter 6 for more about the effects of meningococcal disease.)

Fever, headache, a stiff neck, and pain looking at bright light are the most common symptoms. Some people may have a red rash as well as nausea, vomiting, and lightheadedness. Long-term effects can include brain damage, deafness, limb amputation, or kidney damage.

Because meningococcal disease can be spread through close contact, such as living or going to school in close quarters or kissing, the first dose is given by age 12, with a booster given at age 16.

TECHNICAL STUFF

The vaccine gets its name from the fact that it protects against many of the most common types of meningococcal bacteria, but not all of them. It does protect against A, C, W, and Y, four serotypes of meningococcus. A separate vaccine, given in adolescence, protects against type B.

REMEMBER

Your child may complain of a sore arm or muscle aches after this vaccination. Talk to your doctor if your child has had a severe allergic reaction to any of the components of the vaccine.

Tetanus, diphtheria, and pertussis (Tdap)

Like the DTaP vaccine given to infants and young children (covered earlier in this chapter), the Tdap vaccine protects against diphtheria, tetanus, and pertussis. The difference is that the Tdap, given to children over age 7, contains a smaller dose of the antigens for diphtheria and pertussis (also called whooping cough). This is considered a booster shot and is given between age 11 and 12.

TIP

After this vaccination, your child can wait ten years until their next booster of Tdap. Children who are accident prone and have a tendency to accidentally puncture or otherwise injure themselves regularly may need a booster repeated at five years. You can expect to be asked, "When was my last tetanus shot?" if your child is prone to stitches, since every healthcare provider who sews him back up will ask.

Needing a Booster: Vaccines for Teens

The vaccines for teens are nearly all repeat, or booster, injections (see Table 8-5).

TABLE 8-5

Vaccines for Teens at a Glance

Vaccination	Age Given
Influenza	Yearly
MenACWY	Age 16

Here's the scoop on a few specific vaccines for teens:

>> **HPV:** If your teen didn't start the HPV series before age 15, they will need three doses to complete the vaccination. The second dose should be given one to two months after the first, and the third six months after that. (We introduce the HPV vaccine earlier in this chapter.)

>> **MenACWY (and maybe MenB):** The booster shot for meningococcal disease, MenACWY, is given at age 16. Because the first dose, given at age 11 or 12, will wear off over time, it's important for teens to get the booster before they head off to areas where meningococcal diseases can spread quickly, like college dorms, military living quarters, or just renting a one-room apartment with ten of their closest friends.

In some cases, your doctor may also recommend your teen age 16 or older getting the vaccine against three serotype B, called MenB, strains. These are less common than other types of meningococcal disease, but outbreaks have occurred at some colleges. Several doses of MenB are needed to confer immunity, and the vaccinations must be the same brand. Different brands require a different number of boosters, and the timing varies. Talk to your healthcare provider about the specific number of injections needed.

TIP

Some teens, more often girls, may become anxious about vaccines. They may even pass out after being vaccinated. Have your teen stay seated (or even lie down if feeling dizzy) for a few minutes after the vaccination if you're worried about them fainting afterwards.

Catching Up on Childhood Vaccines

Sometimes you end up having to play catch-up with your child's vaccinations. Maybe you started vaccinations late because of a health issue, or maybe you wanted to spread out the vaccinations, with your healthcare provider's approval. If you've adopted a child from overseas, you may also find yourself needing to catch up on vaccinations not commonly given in other countries.

Spreading vaccines out

If you spread out your child's initial vaccines because you were concerned about giving too many vaccines at once, it's never too late to get back on schedule. (Hopefully, we've reassured you in this chapter that the current vaccination schedule is safe for your child.)

It's usually the infant vaccination schedule that gets modified if parents are concerned about the number of injections given at time. Some healthcare providers offer a slow vaccine schedule that still covers your baby's initial vaccinations and catches up by the time they hit toddlerhood. While some of these catch-up schedules have been widely published, it's important to know that they're not endorsed by the American Academy of Pediatrics, the Center for Disease Control, or the American Academy of Family Physicians.

REMEMBER

It's also important to remember that if your children develop any of the illnesses the vaccines are designed to prevent, they will be exposed to far more antigens than they would be from the vaccine. And worse, they will be exposed to potential complications that can cause far more harm than a vaccine. We address the myths and misconceptions of vaccines and vaccine schedules in more detail in Chapter 11.

Starting vaccines late

Occasionally, parents decide not to vaccinate their child and then change their mind. Obviously, we're all for changing your mind and deciding to have your child vaccinated. An outbreak of a disease in your area may have you second-guessing your original decision. Or your child may have had a serious illness that interrupted their vaccination schedule.

REMEMBER

In most cases, the best thing to do is to start your child's schedule at the beginning. Skipping doses or skipping certain vaccines isn't advised unless your healthcare provider recommends doing so.

Adopting a child from another country

When you're adopting a child from another country, you don't have much say in their vaccination schedule or their exposure to disease before they arrive at your home. Your agency may have no information about your new child or any type of health records. Over 90 percent of internationally adopted children are behind on their vaccinations upon their arrival.

Many adopted children come from countries where certain diseases, such as hepatitis A, are endemic. Not only do you have to worry about your new child getting sick, but you also have to worry that they may spread illness to you or other family members.

TIP

One thing you can and should do is to make sure that all your current family members — including great grandma and grandpa — are up to date on their own vaccinations.

Some international agencies will try to get started on some immunizations before your new family member comes home. International adoptions are rarely fast; they're a fairly drawn-out process that involves making sure no one comes for the child, or that the child is ready to be adopted. Sometimes it takes a while for the right family to be found. During that time, a good agency will get basic immunizations started.

However, many countries don't vaccinate at all against diseases such as hepatitis A or common childhood illnesses such as chicken pox, measles, mumps, or rubella, so your child will still likely be behind on vaccinations.

Healthcare providers may test for antibodies to see whether your child has immunity to common diseases. They may also recommend that you start the immunization schedule as if your newest family member had no immunity to any diseases.

Checking Out Vaccine Schedules Around the World

TIP

Every country creates its own pediatric vaccine schedule. In some countries, diseases that have been eliminated in other countries are still very common. Numerous factors can affect a country's vaccine schedules, including lack of availability in some areas. The World Health Organization maintains a current list of every country's vaccination schedules at apps.who.int/immunization_monitoring/globalsummary.

For the most part, vaccination schedules in Europe and most developed countries are quite similar to the United States' vaccination schedule. Vaccines may be given at different ages and in different doses, but with a few exceptions, the overall schedule is quite similar.

Chapter **9**

Vaccines for Adults

The need for vaccinations doesn't just disappear when you reach the magic age of 18. But the schedule does begin to spread out once you reach adult-hood. In fact, it can be easy to forget about vaccinations when you're busy working, moving a few times, and raising kids and worrying about *their* vaccination schedules. Things don't get any easier when you get older, as you try to juggle your parents' needs, your adult children's crises, and your own increasing health concerns.

Your own health needs may take a back seat to things like job promotions, buying houses, and going to your kid's soccer games. But you need to keep yourself healthy, and that really does mean making a yearly pilgrimage to your own healthcare provider's office and keeping yourself on track with your own vaccinations.

Vaccines When You're 19–26 Years Old

These are the years where you're most likely to be living in crowded conditions, whether it be a college dorm, military barracks, or an apartment with an ever-changing array of roommates and their friends. Because some diseases spread easily in crowded conditions like these, it's important to be up to date on vaccinations.

Yes, it sounds like such a kid thing — and you're not a kid anymore — but part of being an adult means making good choices for your own health. So the following sections cover what you need, vaccine-wise, to keep yourself healthy during the years when sleep, good eating habits, and other health measures may go out the window.

REMEMBER

If you're up to date on all your vaccinations from childhood (see Chapter 8), the list is actually quite short. If you haven't had all the recommended doses up to this point, talk to your healthcare provider about getting back on track. Some people aren't vaccinated for HPV (human papillomavirus), especially men, but also some women. You're eligible to be vaccinated, and the vaccine does help prevent HPV-related cancers and genital warts. Others may have missed the meningococcal vaccine but are now living in a crowded setting; it's important then to make sure you're vaccinated for meningococcus.

Your yearly flu shot

The flu shot is the one vaccination that never ends. Year after year, the news and billboards will remind you, and your healthcare provider will ask every year, "Have you had your flu shot?" When you're young, a flu shot may not seem like much of a priority. Few young adults die from the flu, after all, so why worry?

While it's true that death rates from the flu are low in the 19- to 26-year-old age group, the flu takes an enormous toll on people — and on the economy, when thousands of people miss work over the winter. And while a week off work may sound okay, the flu really isn't much fun. It also can spread to others who aren't so lucky to bounce back from it.

Lots of people say they had the flu when what they actually had was some other virus, maybe one with a little sniffly nose or some nausea. That's not the flu. When you have the flu, you can expect

>> Fever, lasting maybe up to a week

>> Headache

>> Muscle aches that make you feel like you can't even get out of bed

>> Cough that usually keeps you up all night

>> Sore throat

REMEMBER

In other words, when you have the flu, you're sick. Like, really sick. And not only are you sick, but you're also contagious. Which means people to whom the flu can be very dangerous can catch it from you, like kids and older adults.

There are two versions of the influenza vaccine: the live attenuated vaccine, given as a nasal spray, and an inactive vaccine, given as an injection. The nasal spray vaccine is not always available, but when it is, most adults can get either form of the vaccine.

You should not get the live influenza vaccine if

>> You're over the age of 50.

>> You have a severe allergy to any of the ingredients in the vaccine.

>> You're pregnant.

>> You have a compromised immune system.

>> You live with or care for someone with a compromised immune system.

>> You have cochlear implants.

>> You don't have a spleen.

>> You have an active cerebrospinal fluid leak.

>> You took an antiviral medication for the flu, within the previous 48 hours for oseltamivir and zanamivir, within the previous 5 days for peramivir, or within the previous 17 days for baloxavir (these are all different types of antiviral medications).

The live flu vaccine does *not* give you the flu, but it can cause mild side effects, including headache, cough, or runny nose. Breastfeeding moms can take either the live or inactive flu vaccine.

The COVID-19 vaccine

Since we're still working on the first round of COVID-19 vaccines at the time of this writing, it's hard to say whether or not this will turn into an annual vaccination. But at this point, it's fair to say that none of us wants to go through another year like 2020, so if a yearly vaccination does become available, you should get it. Although death rates from COVID-19 are still fairly low the 19-26 age group, they're not as low as they are from the flu.

Because this disease is still evolving so much, it's almost impossible to determine what will happen next. Symptoms of COVID-19 can include the following:

>> Fever

>> Muscle aches

>> Headache

>> Sore throat

>> Loss of taste or smell

>> Congestion

>> Fatigue

We discuss the most up-to-date information available on COVID-19 in Chapter 3.

A Tdap or Td booster

Tdap stands for tetanus, diphtheria, and pertussis, or whooping cough. Td is often given as a booster to adults but leaves out the pertussis portion. It's important that pregnant women get the Tdap vaccine during each pregnancy. (We discuss pregnancy later in this chapter.)

REMEMBER

It's also important that anyone who will be around small babies — grandma, big sister, or uncle, for example — is also vaccinated with the Tdap vaccine. The CDC recommends the Tdap shot for anyone who expects to have close contact with an infant younger than 12 months old. It's best to have a Tdap if you anticipate having any contact with infants.

Any adult who has not had Tdap should be vaccinated with this as an adult at least once to try to stop the spread of pertussis. If you were vaccinated on time as a child, you last had this vaccination when you were 11 or 12. It's good for ten years, so you need a booster at 21 or 22. You may need it sooner if you step on a rusty nail, have a dirty wound, or need stitches. In that case, you need a vaccine if you have not had one in the last five years.

Tetanus remains a threat worldwide. About 1 million people develop tetanus because they are not properly vaccinated. It is thought that close to 40,000 die from tetanus each year. It's a horrible disease, as it can cause a slow suffocation, with shallow breaths and lots of painful body spasms.

Tetanus isn't common in the United States anymore since the advent of the vaccine. One hundred years ago, it used to be that a game of football (whether American football or soccer) carried a small but real risk of tetanus for which there wasn't a vaccine or treatment. Nowadays, the cases of tetanus that do happen usually occur in adults who either haven't ever had the vaccine or haven't kept up with their boosters. Those with diabetes and chronic wounds are at greater risk. Some countries only require vaccination in childhood alone, but the Centers for Disease Control (CDC) recommends getting the booster every ten years.

Diphtheria, which can cause breathing problems, heart failure, or death, has been almost completely eliminated in the United States, with fewer than five cases reported in the last ten years. Most cases are related to travel from areas where the bacteria is still spreading. Vaccination has prevented these cases from spreading to others. The CDC recommends this booster every ten years.

Vaccines When You're 27–49 Years Old

REMEMBER

Although your life has undoubtedly changed quite a bit over these two decades, your immunization schedule has stayed pretty much the same. You need the same three vaccines that you needed in your early to mid-twenties, as we discuss earlier in this chapter: influenza every year, Td every ten years, and possibly COVID-19 vaccinations.

On average, between 5 and 20 percent of Americans catch the flu each year. If you don't get the flu shot, the average number of work days missed because of the flu is between three and seven days. And in this age group, you're likely to either have young children or be helping with elderly relatives, the two age groups most susceptible to complications from the flu.

Do catch up on the HPV vaccination as well if you were not vaccinated when you were younger. The earlier you're vaccinated, the earlier you're protected from acquiring new strains of HPV (up to nine in the vaccine).

Vaccines When You're 50–64 Years Old

REMEMBER

In addition to the influenza, COVID-19, and tetanus vaccines, there's a very important newcomer to your vaccine schedule once you hit age 50: the shingles (recombinant zoster) vaccine. This vaccine, given in a two-shot series, protects you against herpes zoster, better known as shingles. This is the virus that you got when you had chicken pox as a kid, and the virus has been sleeping in your nerve roots ever since. It can crop out when you least want it, causing a limited but quite painful bubbly rash on one side of your body.

Starting at age 50, you're eligible for the shingles vaccine (brand name Shingrix). This vaccine provides protection against shingles for 97 percent of recipients. It also protects 91 percent of people against a painful long-term complication called postherpetic neuralgia (PHN). PHN can cause chronic nerve pain that can be very difficult to eradicate.

You don't have to sign up for the vaccine on your 50th birthday; you can get it any time after you turn 50. But the sooner the better. A single episode of shingles is extremely painful, while PHN can cause years of misery.

REMEMBER

If you've had chicken pox, you're at risk for developing shingles at some point in your life. The virus that causes chicken pox remains in your body and can cause an outbreak of shingles any time later in life. Around 33 percent of people who've had chicken pox will develop shingles at some point, and it's estimated that 99 percent of people born before 1980 have had chicken pox, whether they remember it or not. It's best to be vaccinated even if you don't remember having chicken pox.

You can also be vaccinated for shingles if you have had the chicken pox vaccine; shingles can develop from the live chicken pox vaccine, though this is pretty rare. Ten percent of people who have shingles develop PHN, and you really want to avoid this.

You'll need two doses of the Shingrix vaccine, spaced two to six months apart. If for some reason you don't get your second vaccination within six months, get it as soon as you can. You don't have to start the series over.

This is a reactogenic vaccine, meaning you'll feel your immune system getting to work. The injections are given into the muscle of your upper arm. Shingrix is an inactive vaccine. The most common side effects in clinical trials include

>> Muscle soreness in 44 percent

>> Fatigue in 44 percent

>> Headache in 37 percent

>> Shivering in 26 percent

>> Fever in 20 percent

>> Gastrointestinal issues in 17 percent

You *should* get the shingles vaccine if

>> You're over age 50. There's no upper age limit.

>> You've had Zostavax, an older shingles vaccine, in the past.

>> You've already had shingles. Even if you've had shingles in the past, the vaccine can help protect you in the future.

You *should not* get the shingles vaccine if

>> You've had a severe reaction to any ingredient in the vaccine.

>> You want protection from chicken pox.

>> You have never had chicken pox, you test negative, and you were born after 1980. In this case, you should get the chicken pox, or varicella, vaccine. (However, if you were born before 1980, you've almost certainly had chicken pox even if you or your family members don't remember having it. You should skip the chicken pox vaccine and be vaccinated for shingles at 50, as there's a 99 percent chance you've had chicken pox and need protection from shingles.)

>> You currently have shingles.

>> You are currently pregnant or breastfeeding.

>> You're currently ill or have a fever greater than 100.3 degrees Fahrenheit.

Vaccines When You're 65-Plus Years Old

The retirement age brings with it a new designation: elderly. You may not feel elderly, and you may not look it either, but at age 65, this is how you're classified. While it brings some good things, like discounts on haircuts and grocery store bills, it also can bring a rise in annoying or serious health issues. Like it or not, things change as you get older; your immune system isn't as effective at protecting you from diseases, and that can increase your need for immunizations.

Influenza

You've been hearing for years how important it is to get your yearly influenza vaccination. And if you've been kind of forgetting to get it every year up until now, it's time to turn over a new leaf. Flu complications take a large upward turn over age 65, with between 70 and 85 percent of deaths from flu and between 50 and 70 percent of hospitalizations from flu occurring in people over 65.

Knowing the risks

You may think that your risks of getting the flu are low; maybe you don't go out all that much, or you feel that because you don't have any known lung issues, you'll be able to weather the flu if you do get it. Wrong on both counts. The common risks of the flu are well known, but there are also hidden risks to getting the flu over age 65.

You have a higher risk of developing complications from the flu when you're over age 65 if you suffer from any of the following:

>> Chronic lung disease such as asthma, chronic obstructive pulmonary disease (COPD), or lung cancer

>> Diabetes

>> Heart disease

>> Immune disorders

>> Kidney disease

>> Liver disease

>> Obesity, particularly if you have a body mass index (BMI) over 35

You may know that one of the main risks of having the flu when you're over 65 is an increased risk of developing pneumonia. You also are at increased risk from blood clotting. What you may not know is this:

>> Your risk of having a heart attack increases by three to five times in the two weeks after you catch the flu.

>> Your risk of stroke increases by two to three times in the first two weeks after you have the flu.

>> Overall, your risk from dying in the weeks after you have the flu increases sixfold.

Timing your flu shot

October (or the second half of September) is the best time to get the flu shot because it gives your immune system time to develop antibodies (which generally takes a few weeks). The flu season is in full swing between December and February, although cases can occur as early as October and as late as May.

Comparing vaccines for flu over 65

As if things weren't complicated enough, you also need to decide whether you want to take the regular flu shot or the newer flu vaccine created for high-risk people. Your doctor may make this choice for you, but it's always good to understand the reasons behind medical decisions, so talk to your doctor about which is best for you.

You can receive a standard flu vaccine if the vaccine for your age group isn't available. The issue is you likely won't make as many of the antibodies you need (perhaps just 50–75 percent) to protect yourself. You shouldn't, however, have the nasal flu vaccine, which is a live vaccine and isn't recommended for adults 50 and over.

Here's a list of the flu vaccine choices when you're 65 or older:

>> FLUAD (Trivalent) is an inactive, regular-dose flu vaccine with an adjuvant added to increase its effectiveness. This vaccine protects against three flu strains: two A and one B. This is the standard flu shot given to people under age 65. (See Chapter 2 for more about flu strains.)

>> FLUAD Quadrivalent protects against four flu strains: two A and two B.

>> FLUZONE High-Dose Quadrivalent is an inactivated, high-dose quadrivalent vaccine with an adjuvant containing four times as much of the antigen. This helps your immune system build antibodies and also protects against four flu strains: two A and two B.

Taking antiviral drugs

If you think you have the flu, antiviral flu drugs, if given soon after symptoms appear, can reduce the number of days that you experience symptoms. These drugs, which are obtained only by prescription, work best when given in the first two days after flu symptoms begin. They may also prevent complications such as pneumonia. It's best, though, to prevent the flu with vaccination.

Tdap

You may forget about updating your Tdap vaccine every ten years. It often comes to people's attention after they puncture themselves with a dirty object and start wondering when their last tetanus vaccination was.

To avoid this, keep a record of your vaccinations and get the vaccine every ten years. Then, every scrape or run-in with a nail won't have you in a panic.

When you're older you're more at risk from tetanus, especially if you have diabetes. You also want to be vaccinated for pertussis (the "p" in Tdap) to avoid giving any baby grandchildren or other babies whooping cough, which can be deadly in small babies.

Pneumococcal vaccines

Two vaccines that protect against not only pneumococcus, a common cause of pneumonia, but also infections in the blood, heart, and around the brain become important once you turn 65. Depending on what medical conditions you have, you may already have had some doses of these vaccines. (Flip to Chapter 6 for an introduction to pneumococcal vaccines.)

REMEMBER

Your doctor can go over which doses you have had before and your medical history, and may recommend different combinations of PCV13 (a pneumococcal conjugate vaccine covering 13 serotypes, also known as Prevnar 13) and PPSV23 (a pneumococcal polysaccharide vaccine of 23 serotypes, also known as Pneumovax 23). If you were a smoker or had diabetes, sickle cell, alcoholism, or immune system issues, you may have had a shot before, but check with your healthcare provider about which dose or doses you need now.

If you have had immune system issues, a cerebrospinal fluid leak, or cochlear implants, you have probably had these vaccines and may need only one more (PPSV23) shot.

If you haven't had any of these vaccines, the CDC recommends both, giving the PCV13 first. They should not be given at the same time and are generally given at least a year apart.

Vaccines Before and During Pregnancy

WARNING

Pregnancy brings a number of new health concerns, and one of them is the need for vaccinations that help protect your baby from certain diseases. While a few vaccinations are recommended during pregnancy, others — particularly live vaccines such as varicella, measles, mumps, and rubella (MMR) — shouldn't be given during pregnancy because of a theoretical risk of the virus spreading to the fetus.

There are also vaccines that are not live vaccines and appear safe, but we recommend being vaccinated, if needed, before pregnancy, as the effects on pregnancy still need to be studied more — such as with HPV and the inactivated shingles vaccine.

Your healthcare provider may recommend checking your blood before you get pregnant to see whether you have antibodies to rubella, a disease that can cause serious birth defects in your baby. If you're not immune, you should get the vaccination at least a month before you get pregnant.

You may also want to see whether you have hepatitis B, which can also harm your newborn. Hepatitis B vaccination is recommended in general. Your healthcare provider may encourage hepatitis B vaccination if

>> Your partner or a close household member has hepatitis B.

>> You've had two or more sexual partners in the last six months.

>> You use intravenous drugs.

>> You have been recently treated for a sexually transmitted disease.

>> You are at high risk at work (healthcare, working with dialysis patients).

REMEMBER

Two vaccines are generally recommended for all pregnant women: the flu vaccine (assuming your pregnancy falls during the flu season) and the Tdap vaccine for tetanus and pertussis, or whooping cough. Both are given to protect you during pregnancy and to protect your newborn baby from both illnesses, which can be especially serious in newborns. Neonatal tetanus used to be a common cause of death and illness for newborns when their umbilical cord stumps became infected. You should have the Tdap vaccine between weeks 27 and 36 of pregnancy. The flu shot can be given in any trimester of pregnancy. You should receive the inactivated flu vaccine, not the live nasal spray during pregnancy.

Pregnant women are especially likely to become more ill if they come down with the flu. The increased risk comes from the fact that your immune system, heart, and lungs all undergo changes that make you more susceptible to complications from the flu.

Vaccines for Travelers

Travel has never been safer, in some respects. But on the other hand, more people than ever are traveling to "exotic" and unusual destinations, having become bored with travel to safe locations. Once travel becomes less restricted due to COVID-19, many people will be flying around the world looking for previously rarely visited countries to go see.

You should have no trouble developing such a list of places to see. But before you do, stop and think of the trouble you get into by not having vaccines to deal with some of the interesting diseases you may run into.

Every area has susceptibility to different diseases that are endemic. You may need to contact your medical provider or the health office in the country of your choice to find out what's required at least six weeks before you prepare to travel out of country. It can take that long to develop immunity to some of the vaccines you'll require. Some may be required; others may be left to your discretion.

The CDC website (wwwnc.cdc.gov/travel/) has a complete list of what vaccines are required in different countries as well as a list of how to find centers that give certain vaccines.

Making sure you're up to date on routine vaccines

While you're checking up on what vaccines you need to travel to exotic locales, don't forget to make sure you've kept your routine vaccines up to date. If you're exposed to something in the middle of nowhere, it may not be easy to get vaccinated on the fly, and vaccines take a couple of weeks to work even if you can find someone to vaccinate you.

Some diseases, such as measles and chicken pox, have become uncommon in the United States but aren't routinely vaccinated against even in parts of Europe, in part because of concerns over vaccines. And it's much easier to just get a tetanus booster before you leave if you don't know when your last one was than to try to find one after you've punctured yourself with something in the middle of a jungle somewhere. Do make sure you are up to date on your flu vaccine, as this is a common cause of illness with travel.

Getting other vaccines depending on your destination

There's one vaccine you may need to take in order to be allowed to enter some countries — the yellow fever vaccine. There are specific countries where yellow fever transmission is a worry, and so travelers are required to show they are vaccinated and not introducing the virus. This is true especially if you are traveling from another country where yellow fever can be found. This applies to parts of Africa and South America. Yellow fever can cause outbreaks, transmitted from person (or monkey) to person by mosquitoes. It can cause symptoms ranging from fever, jaundice, chills, and body aches to organ failure.

Yellow fever vaccines are given only in certain centers in the United States, and you may have to travel to find one. One dose of the live vaccine is now thought to confer lifelong immunity, though previously you needed to get a booster every ten years.

Consider the following vaccines as well:

WARNING

>> Do make sure you have vaccinations for typhoid and hepatitis A as well if you may be traveling in an area where this may be a risk. Both spread through contaminated water or food, especially if handled by someone who is currently infected, or through unwashed hands from fecal-oral contact.

Typhoid is a bacterial infection that can cause serious fevers as well as a gastrointestinal infection that should be treated with antibiotics. Hepatitis A is a type of viral liver infection that can cause you fatigue, yellowing eyes or skin, abdominal pain, fever, and diarrhea.

>> If you weren't vaccinated before for hepatitis B, it's always best to be vaccinated, especially if you may ever be sexually active, work in a health facility, or be hospitalized while traveling.

>> If you travel to some parts of West Africa, it's best to be vaccinated for meningococcus meningitis because regular outbreaks of meningitis can occur in the dry season.

>> If you might be around wild dogs, bats, or other wildlife where there is rabies, discuss with your provider whether you should have a rabies vaccine. Rabies isn't found everywhere (it's not in Australia, New Zealand, Great Britain, or Hawaii), but there are areas where it is more common. Rabies is a virus that can cause a serious brain infection that is usually deadly, but it can be prevented if you are vaccinated beforehand or immediately after exposure.

REMEMBER

If you are bitten by a dog or another animal that may have rabies or have an exposure to bats where there may be rabies, it's important to see a medical provider right away (that same day) to start a series of vaccines for rabies and maybe receive an injection of immunoglobulins (antibodies) if you haven't been vaccinated. Being vaccinated ahead of time makes it safer for you when traveling in rural areas where it would be hard to seek medical care immediately after exposure to a rabid animal. This is especially important if you are camping, exploring caves, working with animals, or spending a lot of time in rural areas where dog exposures are common.

If you have been vaccinated ahead of time, you still need to get your vaccinations right away, though you don't need the immunoglobulins and you won't need so many doses (just on day 0 and day 3). If you haven't been vaccinated before, you'll need four doses (day 0, day 3, day 7, day 14) and immunoglobulins.

>> If you're traveling through East Asia, you may need the Japanese encephalitis vaccine. Like yellow fever, this is a mosquito-borne disease that kills 20 to 30 percent of its victims and leaves between 30 and 50 percent of survivors with serious neurological effects.

>> The cholera vaccine, given as a single oral dose of a live vaccine, can give you immunity for three to six months (or maybe longer). It is not available in the United States now, but there are other vaccines, which are oral and inactivated. Cholera is transmitted via the oral-fecal route and spreads through contaminated food, water, or sewage. If you're traveling through certain parts of the Caribbean, Africa, and/or Southeast Asia, talk to your doctor about taking this vaccine. Drinking bottled water only, even to brush your teeth, and eating only cooked foods can help you avoid this infection.

REMEMBER

>> Don't forget malaria prophylaxis. Malaria is an infection that can cause terrible fevers; low blood counts; and kidney, lung, and brain issues if you're bitten by the wrong mosquito. It's best to avoid this. A malaria vaccine for kids is being studied and rolled out in some countries. No vaccine is licensed in the United States for malaria, and scientists are still looking for one that works well in adults. In the meantime, you'll need to take a pill before you go, while you're away, and after you return to make sure you stay safe from malaria. So make sure you check in with your doctor well before traveling so you are all set.

Catching Up: If Your Parents/Guardians Didn't Vaccinate You

REMEMBER

It's never too late to catch up on vaccinations. If your parents or guardians didn't have you vaccinated or skipped some vaccines, it's not too late. If you decide to catch up on vaccines as an adult, it's not really that difficult. The CDC website at www.cdc.gov/vaccines/schedules/downloads/adult/adult-combined-schedule.pdf lists which vaccines should be given if you're just getting started with your vaccinations as an adult.

Chapter **10**

Spelling Out Who May Face Risks

While vaccines have numerous benefits, there are times when you may be advised not to take one. On the other hand, you may think you should not be vaccinated because of an allergy or health condition, but it may be totally fine to do so. This chapter explains when vaccines are safe and when you're better off to wait or avoid a certain vaccine altogether.

Knowing When to Avoid or Limit Vaccines

REMEMBER

Vaccinations are most effective when your immune system is strong enough to generate a response to them. When your immune system is weakened, either by disease or by treatments you're undergoing, the vaccine may not produce the desired effect — immunity to the disease the vaccine is meant to protect against.

The following sections discuss instances when vaccines may need to be avoided or timed differently.

Considering vaccines and cancer

Not all cancer treatments weaken your immune system, but some certainly do. Those who require chemotherapy, radiation therapy, prolonged steroid use, bone marrow or organ transplant, or immunologic therapy or anti-B cell therapy certainly should talk to their doctors about any vaccinations.

Cancer treatments such as chemotherapy and radiation can be a bit of a double-edged sword when it comes to vaccinations. On one hand, the treatment weakens your immune system, making you more susceptible to getting sick. But your weakened immune system also makes it more difficult for you to develop a response to the vaccination that's strong enough to produce immunity.

The following sections give general information on vaccine timing and types when you're being treated for cancer.

Gauging general vaccine timing

The answer to the problem is to have any necessary vaccinations before you begin cancer treatment. This is why you should always be up to date on your vaccines as cancer never gives us any warning. Inactive vaccines usually take two weeks to produce a strong immune response, so talk to your healthcare provider about which ones you may need and schedule them at least two weeks before your treatment begins. Live vaccines should be given at least four weeks before beginning treatment.

It's always good to be up to date on your flu vaccine, and do make sure you're vaccinated for COVID-19, even if you're not in need of any other vaccines.

If you miss this window, you may need to wait until after treatment, and sometimes you need to give your immune system three months to recover to make a strong immune response. If you need to have your spleen removed for leukemia or lymphoma or any other reason, it is best to start vaccinations as soon as possible (possibly starting up to 10–12 weeks before surgery), but hopefully at least two weeks before surgery with vaccines needed to keep you safe once you no longer have your spleen protecting you. If you need to have emergency surgery, you can be vaccinated after; be sure to ask your healthcare provider about this.

Regarding specific vaccine types

Live vaccines are made from a weakened (or related and mild) virus or bacteria. They won't cause disease if your immune system is healthy. Problem is, these same viruses and bacteria can cause an infection if the immune system can't hold them back. They are pretty weak, though, and many live vaccines can be used with immune systems that are mildly weakened.

Live vaccines include varicella (chicken pox); certain zoster (shingles) vaccines; measles, mumps, and rubella vaccines; as well as some travel vaccines, including the yellow fever vaccine. Live vaccines should be avoided altogether once treatment begins unless your healthcare provider recommends them. The current shingles vaccine, Shingrix, is an inactivated vaccine.

WARNING

Influenza is particularly dangerous for people with cancer; between 9 and 33 percent of those who get the flu develop flu complications such as pneumonia. If you're undergoing cancer treatment, the following issues should be discussed with your doctor:

» You should not be given the nasal (FluMist) vaccine, because it's a live vaccine.

» Family members can be vaccinated while you're undergoing treatment with the injection, not the nasal vaccine.

» You can be given the vaccine two weeks before, two weeks after, or between chemotherapy treatments (or later if you've had a more suppressive treatment).

» If you have certain types of blood cancer, such as leukemia or multiple myeloma, you may have a decreased immune response to the flu vaccine.

If you haven't been vaccinated against pneumococcal or meningococcal infections, your doctor may recommend these vaccines before your treatment begins. If you haven't had a recent booster against the Tdap (tetanus, diphtheria, and pertussis) vaccine, your doctor may recommend that as well.

REMEMBER

It's incredibly important now if you have cancer to be vaccinated for COVID-19. If you're actively undergoing treatment or have complications such as decreased blood counts after treatment, talk to your doctor about how to best time the vaccine and treatments to make sure you are protected.

It's also possible that your immune system won't react as well to the vaccine because of the medications you take, giving you slightly less protection than if your immune system were working optimally. Because some protection is better than none, the vaccine is important, and you and your doctor together can decide when to get the vaccine.

Vaccines and immune disorders

Autoimmune disorders affect around 5 percent of the world's population. People with chronic immune disorders such as multiple sclerosis, rheumatoid arthritis, systemic lupus erythematosus, and nearly 100 other types of autoimmune disease have immune systems that have turned against themselves.

In addition, many take medications to calm their immune response, such as high-dose steroids, immunosuppressants, and drugs that decrease tumor necrosis factor, a protein that causes inflammation. This can be a double-edged sword when it comes to vaccinations. It is always best to be fully vaccinated in case you ever get sick in the future and best to be fully vaccinated before starting immunosuppressive treatment.

REMEMBER

Inactivated vaccines are generally safe for use if you have an immune disorder. Talk to your healthcare provider about which vaccines you may need and how they should be timed around treatments.

REMEMBER

Live vaccines should be discussed with your doctor. For a short time, you may need to avoid close family members who get live vaccines as well, such as babies who have had the rotavirus or oral polio vaccine.

Vaccines after organ transplantation

In 2020, transplant teams performed nearly 40,000 solid organ transplants in the United States alone, which include heart, kidney, liver, lungs, and pancreas. The vast majority of patients continue to take immunosuppressive drugs for the rest of their lives, which prevent the body from rejecting the new organ.

REMEMBER

Because immunosuppressive medications weaken the immune system, they increase the risk of developing infection. Most transplant patients can take inactivated vaccines three months after transplant; the influenza vaccine can be given a month after transplant. As with other immunosuppressed people, live vaccines should be avoided.

Because it's not possible for a transplant patient to stop immunosuppressive drugs, they're likely to have a less robust response to vaccinations. If possible, completing vaccinations at least two weeks before transplant surgery will provide the best immunity. This may require starting courses of any vaccines that you are not up to date with a couple of months beforehand. This is possible if the transplant organ is coming from a live known donor, so that surgery can be scheduled, but less possible if the transplant is urgent.

COVID-19 and flu vaccination remain really important for anyone who has an organ transplant.

WARNING

Children who have undergone solid organ transplants pose a special risk because so many common children's vaccines, such as chicken pox, measles, mumps, and rubella, are live vaccines, normally cause a weakened version of the disease. A child on immunosuppressants can become more seriously ill from a live vaccine. If at all possible, live vaccines should be given several weeks before transplant surgery, even if they need to be given before the recommended age.

Family members, including pets, can and should receive all recommended inactivated vaccines. Follow your transplant team's recommendations for live vaccines and close family members.

Understanding Vaccines and Allergies

Many vaccines can cause some type of reaction, including soreness at the site, fever, rash, or generally feeling unwell. These aren't allergic reactions and don't mean that you can't receive the vaccine in the future. However, some vaccine ingredients can cause an allergic reaction, although they may not be the ones you think. The following sections give you the scoop. See Chapter 7 for details on vaccine ingredients and side effects.

REMEMBER

In one U.S. study, just 33 people had a serious allergic reaction to a vaccine out of 25 million vaccinations given. None died, and only one needed hospitalization. Severe allergic reactions rarely occur more than four hours after a vaccine. Delayed reactions such as fever or rash are more likely to be due to your body forming an immune response — a desired response — to the vaccine.

Allergies to vaccine ingredients and components

Antibiotics used in small amounts in some vaccines to keep them from becoming contaminated can cause an allergic reaction. Antibiotics may be used in the manufacturing process to avoid contamination and then removed, but trace amounts may remain.

Some vaccines also contain ingredients that can cause an allergic reaction in susceptible people. Proteins, including egg, yeast, and especially gelatin, tend to cause most allergic reactions.

Antibiotics

Vaccines don't use the antibiotics most likely to cause an allergic reaction — cephalosporins, penicillin, and sulfa drugs. Antibiotics used in vaccines — gentamicin, neomycin, polymyxin B, and streptomycin — are far less likely to cause an allergic reaction. Only one case of an immediate hypersensitivity reaction to neomycin after vaccination has been reported. These antibiotics are sometimes in eye and ear drops and topical antibiotics used on cuts and scrapes.

The vaccines that contain the single antibiotic neomycin include

>> Hepatitis A, B

>> Imovax (rabies)

>> MMR

>> MMRV

>> Varicella

Vaccines that contain several antibiotics include

>> Diphtheria, tetanus, pertussis, polio: Neomycin, polymyxin B

>> Diphtheria, tetanus, pertussis, hepatitis B, polio (Pediarix): Neomycin, poly-myxin B

>> Influenza: May contain gentamicin, kanamycin, neomycin, polymyxin B, or no antibiotics, depending on the manufacturer

>> Polio: Neomycin, polymyxin B, streptomycin

Adjuvants, preservatives, and stabilizers

Ingredients such as adjuvants, which create a stronger immune response, preser-vatives, or stabilizers can also cause a reaction. Oils such as peanut or corn oils — common sources of allergic reactions, especially in children — aren't used in vaccines. However, one vaccine — the flu vaccine used for adults over 65 — does contain shark liver oil (squalene).

WARNING

Gelatin made from bovine or porcine skin and bones is used as a stabilizer in some vaccines. This is one of the most common causes of allergic reactions. Because it contains proteins, it can cause an allergic reaction. Talk to your healthcare pro-vider if you have a severe gelatin allergy to see whether a serum-specific IgE test or skin prick test is necessary. Vaccines that contain gelatin in minute amounts include

>> Live attenuated flu vaccine (FluMist)

>> MMR

>> MMRV (ProQuad)

>> Varicella

Yeast proteins can theoretically cause allergic reactions, although this is rare. Of 180,000 allergic reports in the Vaccine Adverse Event Reporting System, only 15 appeared to result from a reaction to yeast proteins in the vaccines, and even in those cases, it wasn't proven that yeast was the culprit. Vaccines that contain yeast include

>> Hepatitis B vaccines

>> Combination vaccines that include hepatitis B

>> Human papillomavirus vaccines

Egg allergies

Egg allergies — although the most common childhood allergy — still affect fewer than one out of one hundred children. Many people who are allergic to eggs believe this allergy makes it impossible to take vaccines. But very few vaccines contain eggs at all, and even those that do, such as many influenza vaccines that are actually grown in eggs, don't necessarily cause an allergic reaction.

The MMR (measles, mumps, rubella) vaccine also contains minute amounts of egg, but not enough to cause an allergic reaction.

REMEMBER

If you or your child has an allergy to egg, your healthcare provider may recommend waiting for longer observation time after receiving the vaccine. The CDC only considers this necessary for those who have severe reactions (not just hives), who should be vaccinated at their physician's office or a hospital or other medical setting.

TIP

You can talk to your allergist and ask about sensitivity testing if there are any questions about what you may have been allergic to in the past before receiving a possibly related vaccine.

Latex allergies

It's almost unheard of for a vaccine to cause an allergic reaction because of latex. However, if you have a severe latex allergy, you should know that some vials and syringes contain rubber latex. Contact allergies, which is what most people with latex allergy have, don't pose a risk. If you just have a mild skin irritation when exposed to latex, this shouldn't be a problem for vaccination.

If you do have a severe latex allergy, with difficulty breathing or anaphylaxis, you should talk to your provider about vaccines supplied in vials or syringes with latex stoppers. Sometimes a work-around can be devised (taking off the stopper to draw up the vaccine), but for some the allergy is severe enough that this won't be enough. Do talk to your medical provider about any latex allergies, especially if you've had any throat, mouth, or lip swelling or tingling or difficulty breathing.

Different types of reactions

WARNING

The allergic reaction we're most concerned about is anaphylaxis. This is a severe allergic reaction that usually begins right after exposure. An anaphylactic reaction can be life-threatening within minutes, although reactions can also occur several hours later. The reactions can include a lot of different symptoms: rash; hives; swelling of the face, lips, or tongue; difficulty breathing; throat tightening; wheezing; vomiting; diarrhea; stomach pain; a sense of impending doom; a drop in blood pressure; and loss of consciousness.

These anaphylactic reactions are usually due to a rapid, immunoglobulin E (IgE) antibody reaction. Outside of vaccination, proteins in certain foods, such as egg, fish, milk, peanuts, shellfish, soy, tree nuts, and wheat, can cause immediate allergic reactions that can affect every part of the body. This type of severe IgE allergic reaction is rare. It can range from one in a million vaccines to 1 in 100,000, depending on which vaccine is used. An anaphylactic reaction requires immediate treatment with epinephrine injection (or an EpiPen).

Not all rashes or skin reactions are IgE reactions. There can be a delayed-type or T-cell–mediated hypersensitivity rash, as we sometimes see a few days after a COVID-19 vaccination. Other immune reactions can also occur, usually within days or weeks.

TECHNICAL STUFF

One such autoimmune reaction to the swine flu vaccine in 1976 caused an outbreak of Guillain-Barré syndrome (GBS). GBS causes nerve damage that can, in a worst-case scenario, require ventilation for a time and in some cases lead to permanent nerve damage. However, the risk of having GBS after the flu or other illness is higher than having it after a vaccination.

There are other types of hypersensitivity reactions, besides anaphylaxis. These reactions can occur several days or more after vaccination. They can include all sorts of different reactions but are usually quite uncommon:

>> Some people have joint pains after some vaccines.

>> Others can have a rash develop hours or maybe a day after the vaccine. This can be a T-cell reaction, such as that which happens with the Moderna

COVID-19 vaccine, which goes away on its own. There's no problem taking another dose later.

» In rare cases, there can be erythema multiforme, often a bull's-eye rash that can involve hands, feet, and other parts of the body.

» Idiopathic thrombocytopenic purpura (ITP) can occur, which is considered an autoimmune reaction against platelets. ITP causes platelet levels to drop, causing thrombocytopenia. This reaction occurs most commonly after MMR vaccination, affecting between 1 and 3 children per 100,000, usually among those vaccinated as 1-year-old toddlers.

Recognizing reactions that actually aren't allergies

Sometimes reactions occur after vaccination that aren't allergic reactions at all. Many of these reactions, such as pain or hard lumps at the vaccination site, aren't considered an allergic reaction.

REMEMBER

Some people may faint after having a vaccine. This is more common in adolescents. It often happens after the regular vaccines given at this age (meningitis, tetanus, and HPV). This response does not seem to be due to an allergy or the vaccine ingredients (these vaccines have very different ingredients). Instead, it seems to be that teenagers are just a bit more prone to fainting. It's important that a medical professional evaluate this and ensure it isn't anything more serious.

In rare cases a skin infection can develop where the needle went through the skin; skin reddens or darkens around the site of a vaccine, but usually it turns out this isn't an infection at all but just a sign of a healthy and robust immune response to the vaccine.

Taking precautions before vaccination

REMEMBER

If you have severe allergies, you should talk to your doctor about them. These allergies may not be a worry at all. Usually your doctor can say that nothing else needs to be done. In some cases, your doctor may want to send you to an allergist if there are any questions, but usually this isn't necessary.

If you have a severe allergic reaction to a vaccine or any of its ingredients, an allergist can see whether it's possible to develop an IgE test to determine whether you are allergic to the vaccine.

TIP

If you've had previous reactions that aren't allergic reactions, such as swelling, rash, or achiness, take an anti-inflammatory medication such as ibuprofen *after* you take the vaccine. Taking it before can possibly interfere with your body's immune response.

Assessing Reactions to the COVID-19 Vaccine

While there have been some potential allergic reactions to the COVID-19 vaccines, the number of reactions is low. The following sections discuss possible reactions to COVID-19 vaccines and list the ingredients to be aware of.

Rare cases of anaphylaxis

The number of cases of anaphylaxis is small compared to the number of vaccines being given. These occurred more among women and were all treated without more serious issues.

After the first almost 2 million Pfizer vaccines were given, a study found 11.1 cases of anaphylaxis per 1 million. After 4 million doses of the Moderna vaccine, 10 cases of anaphylaxis were seen; this was 2.5 cases per million. Most of these reactions happened within 15 minutes of the vaccine being given.

Those vaccinated are asked to wait 15–30 minutes afterwards to be sure they don't have any symptoms. Only one case of anaphylaxis occurred at 45 minutes after a Moderna shot. There were a few reactions that occurred after 15 minutes with the Pfizer vaccine, but most were under 15 minutes and all were under 2.5 hours.

The U.S. rollout of the Johnson & Johnson vaccine has seen no reported cases of anaphylaxis, but one case was seen in South Africa.

Other types of reactions

Skin reactions are common after vaccines of any type. A lump at the injection site or a rash around the site isn't generally concerning and usually will go away.

The COVID-19 vaccines are considered *reactogenic*. That means they can cause a reaction, an immune response, we can often feel. The result is that we have an immune system trained to fight COVID-19 and we usually feel fine in a day or two.

With the current COVID-19 vaccines that require two injections approximately one month apart, the second injection can cause more of a reactogenic response than the first. Commonly reported symptoms with either the first or second injection include

>> Swelling, redness, and itchiness around the injection site that can occur a few days to up to a week later (called COVID arm)

>> Fever

>> Generalized body aches

>> Fatigue

>> Headache

These reactions aren't considered an allergic reaction. You can get the second vaccine if you have any of these symptoms with the first injection.

Inspecting ingredients found in current COVID-19 vaccines

All vaccines contain ingredients in addition to the part that actually tells your body to create antibodies (see Chapter 5 for details on how vaccines work). You can have a reaction to any of these ingredients. If you've had a reaction to any of them in the past, taking one of the other vaccines may be best for you.

The cause of anaphylaxis from mRNA vaccines is thought to be due to the polyethylene glycol (PEG). This is something we normally call Miralax, the med some folks take for constipation. It's also in a lot of different bottles in our bathrooms — shampoo, toothpaste, deodorant, and cosmetics. This substance is used in the vaccine to make a safe basket for the mRNA to deliver it to our cells without breaking down, as it otherwise would. The mRNA lasts longer when surrounded by fatty cushions created by PEG.

The Pfizer BioNTech COVID-19 vaccine contains the following ingredients:

>> Messenger ribonucleic acid (mRNA)

>> Potassium chloride

>> Monobasic potassium

>> Phosphate

>> Sodium chloride

>> Dibasic sodium phosphate dehydrate

>> Sucrose (sugar)

The Moderna vaccine contains the following ingredients:

>> Messenger ribonucleic acid (mRNA)

>> Lipids, or fatty substances, including SM (sphyngomyelin)-102, polyethylene glycol [PEG] 2000 dimyristoyl glycerol [DMG], 1,2-distearoyl-sn-glycero-3-phosphocholine [DSPC], and cholesterol

>> Tromethamine

>> Tromethamine hydrochloride

>> Acetic acid (vinegar)

>> Sodium acetate

>> Sucrose (sugar)

The newest vaccine to be approved, Johnson & Johnson's Janssen COVID-19 vaccine, differs from the first two approved vaccines in several ways. It requires only one injection. This means you'll be fully protected even if you have a severe allergic reaction to the first injection. Both the Moderna and Pfizer vaccines also contain lipids wrapped around the mRNA, which can be the source of some allergic reactions. This vaccine doesn't, though it has been associated with blood clots and low platelets (which can lead to bleeding), especially in women under 50. It contains the following:

>> Recombinant, replications-incompetent adenovirus type 26 expressing the SARS-COV-2 spike protein (DNA virus rather than mRNA)

>> Citric acid monohydrate

>> Trisodium citrate dihydrate

>> Ethanol

>> 2-hydroxypropyl-β-cyclodextrin (HBCD)

>> Polysorbate 80

>> Sodium chloride

Getting the COVID-19 vaccine after you've had COVID-19

REMEMBER

Having COVID-19 once doesn't necessarily mean that you're permanently immune. Immunity may last for months, possibly longer, but this may depend on individual responses, and we do have less natural immunity against new variants as the virus continues to evolve. It is important to be vaccinated. If you do get the vaccine, you may have more symptoms with your first vaccine than others; it's a reaction similar to those of people getting their second vaccination. Because you may have residual antibodies to the disease, your body will quickly create new, powerful antibodies, which can worsen your reaction to the shots.

Chapter **11**

Anti-Vaxxers and Debunking Myths About Vaccines

We have vaccines to prevent a large number of diseases that previously killed thousands, if not millions, of people, including children. Since we have these tools, you'd think that getting people to take them, or give them to their children, would be a pretty easy sell. But it's not.

More than 10 percent of American parents have questioned the safety of childhood vaccines and the way they're currently given. They may reluctantly vaccinate their children, giving the vaccines on a delayed schedule, giving some but not others, or not giving them at all. In this chapter, we address how this situation started, why it continues in the face of obvious eradication of killer illnesses, and how health-care providers can fight against it.

Studying the Rise of Vaccine Hesitancy

Vaccines save lives. They are studied rigorously both before and after they're released. Before being rolled out to the public, they need to have an excellent record on safety and efficacy. They continue to be studied closely after being released to double-check for any missed complications.

But not everyone wants to be vaccinated or to have their children vaccinated. Some want no vaccines; some hesitate on some vaccines but not others. Some want to space out vaccines, and others accept them but remain uncertain.

REMEMBER

Vaccine hesitancy doesn't mean someone refuses a vaccine. Instead, it includes the refusal or the delay in acceptance of vaccinations despite their availability. Vaccine hesitancy has affected vaccination rates around the world. Delays in vaccinations lead to children being unprotected for longer periods of their vulnerable younger years. Lowered rates of on-time vaccinations can lead to outbreaks. As vaccine rates dip below the levels needed, infections spread.

Some diseases require high rates of vaccination for all of us to be safe. Dropping confidence in vaccines can affect more than just those who are not vaccinated. Measles is highly infectious, for example, so about 95 percent need to be vaccinated to prevent the virus from spreading. This allows the majority to protect the few who aren't personally protected by the vaccine. This includes those who are vulnerable — infants too young to be vaccinated, those with weakened immune systems, and others for whom the vaccine did not induce immunity. Even if childhood vaccines were delayed from infancy to kindergarten, because there are so many children, we would not be able to fully reach herd immunity with the measles vaccine in the United States.

In the following sections, we go over some reasons why people don't vaccinate and give you a brief history of vaccine hesitancy.

Understanding why some people don't vaccinate

Parents and other individuals choose not to vaccinate for a lot of reasons. Sometimes it's a mix of multiple reasons. Some have concerns about the safety of vaccines. Others lack confidence in those studying and distributing the vaccines; they may feel they can't trust medical institutions and professionals due to bad experiences in their own lives or historically in communities to which they belong.

Others are concerned that pharmaceutical companies or government agencies don't have their best interests at heart. Some want to look for natural alternative health solutions or natural preventions. Some, already making decisions about the foods they eat and their lifestyle, want to be in charge of and make all personal health decisions themselves. Some are concerned there may be a religious issue, including the use of animal proteins, fetal cells, or cell media in vaccines, even if religious leaders have not seen a concern. Campaigns by certain organizations, often far-reaching and through social media, can result in reduced vaccination rates. Rumors and misinformation have spread that continue to evolve and affect how people view vaccines.

THE UKRAINIAN MEASLES ISSUE

Ukrainian vaccination rates for measles used to be among the best in the world. Vaccine hesitancy grew, however, in part fueled by online disinformation and internet trolls. Vaccination rates then dropped, as parents chose not to vaccinate their children. It used to be that almost every one-year-old was vaccinated for measles, but over a few years that number dropped to only about one-half. This was followed by a sudden return of measles; previously held back by vaccination, suddenly the floodgates opened. Over the course of a few years, over 100,000 Ukrainians had measles, and a few dozen died, including children. Needed health resources were diverted for measles cases and the outbreaks spread to other countries, including the United States.

Vaccine hesitancy has grown in some parts of the United States. Most one-year-olds in the United States are vaccinated, as intended, for measles, but vaccine hesitancy has sometimes delayed vaccinations. Currently, around 10 percent of children are not vaccinated for measles by age 2 as expected, though only 5 percent remain unvaccinated by age 5.

The problem this creates is that those who choose not to vaccinate often know others who don't as well, causing there to be hotspots for measles to spread. In the mid-2010s some kindergartens had one in five children not vaccinated. Measles started to pick up in California in these hotspots with low vaccination rates among children.

In 2014, 100 measles cases were found in California linked to Disney theme park visits; there, vaccine rates played a role.

Over 90 percent of those who got sick were unvaccinated, were under-vaccinated, or didn't know whether they were vaccinated. More than one out of ten were too young to have been vaccinated and needed to rely on herd immunity for protection but couldn't, given lower rates of vaccination. This outbreak led to the California government taking measures to make it harder for families to opt out of vaccination without a clear medical reason. As a result, vaccine rates rose.

Together, vaccines save lives. To prevent infections from spreading and not just affecting individuals, but also whole healthcare systems strained by outbreaks, it's important to realize we are all in this together. Infectious diseases don't affect just individuals; they affect whole communities. As a whole, we can create firebreaks by ensuring everyone who can be vaccinated is so we protect those too young or whose immune system is weakened who are not protected by vaccines.

Looking at the early anti-vaxxers

Vaccine hesitancy is nothing new. As long as there have been vaccines, some have had concerns. Even before there were vaccines, there were worries about inoculations.

Long before vaccines, inoculation or variolation let parents protect children from smallpox. *Variolation* involved taking infectious material from the arm of one person with smallpox and passing it with a small cut to the arm of someone else who had never had smallpox to protect against future infection. This was a practice around the world from China and India, through to Turkey, many areas in Africa, and remote parts of Europe. It was first introduced to the United States in 1721 by a man named Onesimus from West Africa held in slavery in Massachusetts. It was first introduced to the United Kingdom by Lady Montagu, the wife of the ambassador to Turkey, who had learned the practice from women there and who let her own son be inoculated.

The practice was so widespread because it saved lives and stopped parental heartbreak. The odds were good, but it was also a gamble. Variolation usually caused a mild infection and then a lifetime of immunity, but sometimes it caused a real illness. Of those who had smallpox, 30 percent died, many were scarred, and some were blinded; of those who had variolation, 1 percent to 3 percent died. The odds meant many parents chose variolation, given how common smallpox was.

There were critics, though. Some pointed to the risks; others thought it was unnatural. Although there were religious figures who embraced the practice, others felt diseases were our divine punishment for sins, and we shouldn't try to undo this.

Variolation was an imperfect way to protect against a common cause of death. Eventually, it led to vaccination, first with a virus thought to be cowpox, which was introduced to the public by Edward Jenner in 1796. (Find out more about him in Chapter 12.)

Once there were vaccines, there were those who were against them. Some didn't believe microbes spread disease and thought illness came from bad air. Others didn't want anything that came from animals, like cows, and felt this was unnatural and against their religion.

In the 1800s, laws in the United Kingdom and later the United States made vaccinations free and available to all and then mandated vaccinations against smallpox. This led to others feeling they were being forced to vaccinate, and they felt the government was imposing too many restrictions on those who chose not to vaccinate. There have been anti-vaccine leagues and protests since the 1800s. As vaccinations led to lower rates of smallpox, some felt the disease was less of a worry and did not see the need for vaccination; if rates of vaccination dropped, more were infected and the cycle started again. Later regulations include clauses for conscientious objectors.

Over the years, more vaccines were introduced. Infections that could not be stopped before finally were. Infections such as diphtheria, tetanus, polio, and measles, which kept so many kids from becoming adults, were no longer the dangers they once were. Outbreaks like yellow fever, which had emptied cities and halted travel, became much rarer.

Vaccine hesitancy over the years has included a number of different concerns, as we discuss in the previous section. Some want to make their own health decisions. Some do not trust the medical profession, governments, or companies. Others see vaccines as artificial or not natural.

REMEMBER

We'll say it again: Vaccines save lives. To prevent infections from spreading and affecting not just individuals, but also whole healthcare systems strained by outbreaks, it's important that everyone who can be vaccinated is. Vaccination is our collective firebreak when outbreaks happen.

Debunking Common Vaccine Myths

Medical decisions are always about risks and benefits. Vaccines have been scrutinized so that possible risks are greatly outweighed by benefits. Some vaccines make us feel sick for a day or so; some cause allergic reactions in some people or can be associated with certain adverse side effects. Vaccines are designed to ensure that the benefit always greatly outweighs the risk. The risk of being struck by lightning in a given year is about two in a million. It happens, it makes the news, but it's no reason to avoid going outside.

The following sections debunk a number of common myths about vaccines.

Myth: Diseases were disappearing before vaccines were invented

REMEMBER

We can do a lot of things to prevent diseases from spreading. Vaccines aren't the only way we can prevent diseases, but they are one of the most effective. As we've seen with COVID-19, non-pharmaceutical interventions (such as masking, social distancing, staying outdoors, and having good ventilation) can reduce our risk, but alone they aren't enough to make COVID-19 go away entirely.

Some infections dropped as municipalities improved clean drinking water and sanitation for all. In particular, cholera and typhoid dropped, as did other diarrheal illnesses. Vaccination has helped prevent even more illness and death from these infections and also from others like rotavirus.

New treatments can help make some infections less deadly but can't protect us as well as a vaccine can. We can treat many bacterial infections with antibiotics, but that doesn't undo all the bad effects these infections can cause. It's best to prevent a deadly disease rather than play with fire. Before the Hib vaccine became common (see Chapter 6), pediatric wards filled every winter with seriously ill children. Some would have meningitis and pneumonia, some would die, and some would have lifelong impairments. Once vaccinations came, this became a rare diagnosis. Likewise, we have antibiotics for pneumococcus and meningococcal meningitis and antivirals for influenza, but these treatments don't erase what these infections can cause. These infections can still be deadly even though we have treatment.

Vaccination sent a lot of diseases packing that otherwise caused outbreak after outbreak. Before vaccination, almost every person got measles, and hundreds died in the United States every year, year after year. With vaccination, measles infections dropped quickly. Now few doctors in the United States have even seen a case in their career. Before vaccination, rubella caused outbreaks, leading to millions of infections, including thousands of deaths of infants as well as stillbirths and miscarriages, and many with lifelong effects from the disease. Rubella is now considered eliminated in the Western Hemisphere, thanks to vaccination.

Myth: Vaccines cause serious side effects, illnesses, and death

There are systems that track any side effects, illnesses, or deaths that occur after vaccination. One of these in the United States is the Vaccine Adverse Event Reporting System (VAERS), which is run by the Centers for Disease Control and Prevention (CDC) and the Food and Drug Administration (FDA). It collects information on any adverse event — or side effect or health problem — that occurs after vaccination. The health issue doesn't have to be caused by the vaccine. Anyone, including patients concerned they have been affected by a vaccine, can report an adverse event directly. Healthcare providers are encouraged to report any health event after a vaccine and are required to report certain more serious and specific health issues. The VAERS program follows these reports to identify patterns or concerns that then prompt further investigation.

Manufacturers of vaccines continue to track their usage for any safety issues after a vaccine is rolled out. These include trials that don't rely on others to report issues but instead track individuals from the start. The CDC also works with different clinical health centers and medical research centers to track any safety issues as vaccines are used by the general public.

The bottom line is that the safety of vaccines is taken very seriously. Multiple systems are in place to independently track and identify any issues with vaccines.

Though quite rare, there are certainly allergies to some vaccines, and it's important to pay attention for them and report any allergies to your doctor. There can also be rare side effects, like a drop in platelets that help the blood clot in some children who have the MMR vaccine (for measles, mumps, and rubella), but this rate is far fewer among vaccinated children than those who have natural measles infections.

Again, these risks for a serious vaccination reaction are low. Keep in mind the CDC reports that on average, we have a two-in-a-million chance each year of being hit by lightning, which is not something many of us ever experience or even worry about. Yet this risk is much higher than the risk of a serious vaccine reaction.

The data from these watchdogs, including the VAERS program, are available online and open to the public. So if you ever have any questions, you can look at the data and see for yourself. You can find the VAERS program at vaers.hhs.gov/.

Myth: Kids don't need to be vaccinated so young

Before we had vaccines, losing babies before age 1 was too common. Children too often didn't make it to their fifth birthdays. Vaccines help babies and children, whose immune systems are still developing and for whom every infection is brand-new, survive through what was once a dangerous period. It's really important for those with the least amount of protection to be protected by vaccination. The vaccine provides a cocoon from the dangers of these microbes.

THE FIRST POLIO VACCINE AND THE CUTTER INCIDENT

In the mid-1900s, summers meant polio scares. Parents worried their children might suddenly be paralyzed and not walk again. They worried they might be unable to breathe and be stuck in a metal tube to help them breathe or die from polio.

Hope grew for parents as researchers raced to make a vaccine. In 1955 after a study of 1.3 million children, the official announcement was made: The first polio vaccine had 80 to 90 percent efficacy in preventing paralytic polio. Vaccinations were started to the relief of parents.

A few weeks later, there was a report of a child who was vaccinated who developed paralysis from polio. Then there was another report and then another. The paralysis began in each of these cases in the vaccinated arm, when it usually began in the legs.

Vaccination was halted and the problem investigated, looking at all the vaccine makers. The problem was shown to be associated with only one vaccine maker: Cutter Laboratory in California. It emerged that the lab did not follow the guidelines for fully disenabling or "killing" the polio virus with formaldehyde, and so the vaccine was able to infect children with the virus. As a result, 40,000 children developed polio, 200 had some paralysis, and 10 died.

The investigation led to more testing of vaccines in production and post-production. Vaccine makers were required to test more samples from each vaccine lot and after bottling, and also take other steps to prevent the live virus from making it into a vaccine, such as increasing the amount of time taken to inactivate it, say with formaldehyde.

Vaccination started back up. Although some areas chose not to have vaccination because of what happened, polio vaccination, given how horrible the disease was, remained popular.

This event showed how important it is to monitor for vaccine adverse events in order to find any as quickly as possible and recall any vaccines as needed.

The diseases that vaccines prevent are often those that are the deadliest for the youngest of children. Rotavirus can quickly dehydrate a baby but not an adult. Haemophilus influenzae type b (Hib) used to fill hospitals in the winter with very ill children, but it is usually a mild disease in adults. Pertussis sends newborns to the ICU but is often just an annoying cough for adults. These vaccines are so important for babies because these infections can do so much more harm to them.

THE NATIONAL VACCINE INJURY COMPENSATION PROGRAM AND A NEW POLIO VACCINE

The Cutter Incident (covered in the earlier sidebar "The first polio vaccine and the Cutter Incident") showed that vaccine production, while very much needed, might be halted by lawsuits. A court decision found that the Cutter Laboratory should pay those injured by the polio vaccine. This eventually led the way to streamlining the compensation to anyone who had a serious side effect possibly related to a vaccine.

Since the 1980s, the National Vaccine Injury Compensation Program (www.hrsa.gov/vaccine-compensation/index.html) has provided financial compensation to those who file a petition after having been potentially injured by a vaccine covered by the program (the standard and approved vaccines). This is funded by a small tax on routine childhood vaccines. Even when it's not clear if the vaccine caused the injury, compensation may be provided through a settlement. This program allowed manufacturers to focus on production without continuously responding to potential lawsuits. Such lawsuits against healthcare workers and manufacturers were threatening to cause vaccine shortages. Vaccines are the first medical product that doesn't have direct lawsuits. This covers the routine vaccinations, but as you see in Chapter 13, does not cover permissive recommendations, such as for the Lyme disease vaccine, which was not on the list of routine vaccines and so was not covered.

The Cutter Incident also led us to move from the injectable polio vaccine, which was a killed virus, to the oral vaccine that was later produced and is a live, but weakened, virus. This oral vaccine, the Sabin vaccine, can cause a mild gut infection that can then be shed into the environment, effectively vaccinating others who may drink water contaminated with this virus. The problem is sometimes the virus mutates to a version that can cause actual illness, even very rarely paralysis in someone who is exposed by contact or drinking water. This is called *community circulation of vaccine derived polio virus.*

These cases of vaccine derived polio virus (cVDPV) usually occur in polio type 2. The original, wild-type polio 2 has been eradicated. It was last seen in 1999 and declared eradicated in 2015, but community circulation of vaccine derived polio virus type 2 continues. For this reason, there has been a move to use the injectable vaccines to establish immunity against these type 2 cVDPV cases.

The United States stopped using the oral vaccine entirely in 2000; only the injectable, killed virus vaccine is now used. The oral vaccine continues to be used in low-resource countries where work to eradicate polio continues. Being able to administer the vaccine by drops or on a sugar cube helps make the vaccine feasible. It also helps avoid needles, which require skilled health workers in remote areas and which may be related to vaccine hesitancy for some. Countries that still use the oral type have added the single-dose IPV killed vaccine to create immunity to type 2 without the risk of shedding.

Myth: Kids don't need to be vaccinated when illnesses don't exist in their country

As we have seen with COVID-19, a disease can spread from one side of the world to the other quite quickly. If we don't keep up our collective immunity to an infection, that infection can bounce back very fast.

WARNING

If you aren't vaccinated against an illness, you probably know someone else who isn't vaccinated. These clusters of lower vaccination areas become hotspots where an infection can quickly spread, sometimes before we even realize it. It's not just the risk of you being infected. It's also that you can have an infection that infects someone else who infects someone else who then dies from the illness. You may not even know how your infection affects others. It can be heartbreaking to realize that simple interactions — in a house of worship, in a grocery store, at school — can lead to others dying.

When infections spread, it causes a lot more work for healthcare systems, meaning others who need hospitals for heart attacks or to give birth or after a car accident can't access care easily. There may not be as many health workers who can help, and resources may need to be used to ensure infections don't spread in hospitals. Measles can spread to many more people quickly, if we were not vaccinated or immune, than COVID-19 ever can.

Myth: Giving multiple vaccines at the same time overloads the immune system

REMEMBER

It has been shown that the vaccine schedules, with multiple vaccines at the same time, is safe. (See Chapter 8 for the full scoop on vaccines for children.)

Children today may receive more shots than children in the past, but they actually have fewer immune challenges, or antigens, from vaccines than they did before. They receive far fewer antigens in their first years of life than they did in past decades. Ending smallpox vaccination and switching pertussis vaccination meant no longer having vaccines with 200 or 3,000 antigens, respectively. Instead, a child who is fully vaccinated will have been exposed to a total of 320 antigens by age 2. Real-life infections add up to more exposure to antigens. A case of strep throat itself may have 25–50 antigens; a cold may be 10.

Myth: Vaccines can cause the disease they are supposed to prevent

REMEMBER

As you find out in Chapter 5, most vaccines include only a part of the microbe they're trying to warn against. Sometimes the body's first encounter with this "Wanted" picture of the antigen, along with any adjuvant in the vaccine to strengthen our immune response, can cause a bit of a reaction from our immune system. You may have pain at the site of the vaccine, feel tired or feverish, or have a headache or other symptoms. This usually goes away in a day or two and is a sign of your immune system waking up and making a response to this "Wanted" picture.

We call vaccines that create this response *reactogenic.* Some of the COVID-19 vaccines, as well as the more common zoster vaccine Shingrix and the tetanus vaccines, can cause this sort of reaction. When you feel like you're coming down with the flu after a flu shot, it's not the actual flu; it's usually just your immune system getting ready to protect you from the real flu (unless, of course, you're unlucky enough to have gotten the virus somewhere else before the vaccine can get to work).

Some vaccines include live but *attenuated* — or weakened — virus. These include the MMR (measles, mumps, and rubella), chicken pox, yellow fever, and rotavirus vaccines, as well as the nasal flu vaccine (but not the shot) and the older zoster vaccine (to prevent shingles). These vaccines don't cause the illness they are trying to prevent. We don't administer these live vaccines in pregnancy, but for the most part, it's really only a theoretical risk and not something that's been proven to be a problem.

A few vaccines can cause infections, but they're not the same disease they are preventing:

>> The typhoid oral vaccine uses a weakened version of salmonella bacteria. It can sometimes cause diarrhea or stomach upset that goes away. There's no evidence that it ever changes into anything like the bacteria that causes actual typhoid.

>> The smallpox vaccine (which is rarely given now as the infection has been eradicated around the world) includes another virus, vaccinia. Sometimes, when the vaccine is given, the vaccinated person can spread the vaccinia virus via contact with the vaccine site, which has a little bit of the vaccinia virus. This can lead to skin infections with vaccinia (but not actually smallpox). It can lead to fetal infections as well, so we avoid this in pregnancy.

>> The BCG vaccine (the TB vaccine), which is almost never used in the United States as a vaccination, contains live bacteria, *Mycobacterium bovis,* that is a relative of TB. The vaccine is sometimes used in the United States as treatment for bladder cancer. The BCG is directly inserted by a catheter infusion into the bladder. In rare cases, the bacteria is absorbed into the blood system, spreads, and causes an infection, but it's treatable with tuberculosis treatment (which takes months). This is rare, though, after just a shot of the vaccine. It occurs in less than five in 1 million children and can be quite dangerous and even deadly for small children, who would require TB treatment for months.

>> The oral polio vaccine can also lead to a gut infection with a weakened polio virus. This can shed and spread to others. As long as it remains unchanged, this isn't usually a problem, but in rare cases, it can become an issue. This vaccine has not been used in the United States since 2000.

Myth: Not getting vaccinated affects only me

REMEMBER

Infectious diseases remind us that we are all in this together. The only way we can keep these infections at bay and keep them from disrupting our lives, healthcare, and schooling is to make sure they can't spread in the first place.

If enough of us are vaccinated, we can stop many communicable diseases from spreading at all. This means, though, that a lot of us need to be vaccinated. Some vaccines are more effective than others. Some diseases are more infectious and thus even more people need to be vaccinated to prevent the disease's spread. For some diseases, 19 out of every 20 people need to be vaccinated to stop the spread; other vaccines don't require as much uptake.

We also are vaccinated to protect those around us. Vaccines don't work for everyone. Some people have a weakened immune system and either they can't receive a vaccine or it may not work on them. Others are too young for some vaccines. We want everyone to stay safe.

Myth: Natural immunity is always best

WARNING

Good reasons exist for wanting to avoid the infections that vaccines are created to prevent. These diseases can cause serious damage. For example:

>> Damage can be done to the immune system by natural infections. Measles, for example, can erase our immune system's memory. Many of those "Wanted" photos our immune system has been saving, those antibodies

we've collected over time, are lost when we have measles. The infection erases a lot of our immune memory.

>> Other infectious diseases can cause serious harm — not just death, but also lifelong intellectual impairment, loss of sight and other senses, paralysis, loss of limbs, or other serious side effects we just don't want.

Moreover, natural immunity may just be to one strain, one variant. Vaccines often cover a lot of different strains. We wouldn't want to be infected that many times, let alone once. The HPV vaccine can protect against nine strains. Pneumococcal vaccines protect against as many as 23 strains. We mix in four different types of flu each year, letting us avoid different assortments. It's best to use vaccines to avoid the many different types and strains that can affect us.

Those who are immunocompromised often didn't expect to become that way. You may think you will never have an immune system issue, an autoimmune disease needing immunosuppressive medications, or cancer needing chemotherapy, but this can happen. Medicine can treat a lot of diseases and keep us alive and symptom-free, but these medications may affect our immune system.

Once you're already ill or on immunosuppression, vaccines may not be as effective, so it's important to be vaccinated beforehand. You don't know whether your child will ever have leukemia or Crohn's disease or another medical issue that results in immunosuppression. It's really important that your child does not become sick with a preventable infection when they are most vulnerable.

REMEMBER

One of the worst things to hear as a healthcare provider is a parent saying they thought they were doing what was best for their daughter, as she lies in an ICU bed with a vaccine-preventable illness that her parents decided not to vaccinate her for. It's awful to hear a parent repeating over and over, "But I thought I was doing what was right for her; I thought natural was better."

Myth: The MMR vaccine causes autism

REMEMBER

A large number of studies — hundreds, in fact — have looked for any connection between the MMR vaccine and autism and found none.

The worry started when a publication claimed to show an association between the MMR vaccine and autism. The study looked at a small number of children with developmental regression, including autism, and sought signs of changes in their gut. Most were vaccinated as most children are. The findings were published in 1998 in a well-respected journal, *The Lancet*, and were purported to show that the MMR vaccine and autism were linked. This caused a lot of confusion for parents. Children often are diagnosed with autism at the age when they receive vaccines, and parents worried they might have harmed their child.

The paper that caused all of this confusion about autism and MMR was retracted by the journal in 2010 for fraud. The study did not show that the vaccine caused autism. There have been many studies since then — hundreds, in fact — and again and again they've shown one thing: No connection has been found between the MMR vaccine and autism.

The problem is that many decided to hold off on vaccinating their children for MMR. Consider the following:

>> Measles spread in Europe and in parts of the United States where it was previously unheard of. From 2016 to 2019, measles deaths climbed 50 percent worldwide. Over 200,000 people worldwide lost their lives to measles in 2019.

What's even sadder is that some of those who got measles ended up with the intellectual disabilities that those who were hesitant to be vaccinated were so worried about. We know measles can cause developmental delays and intellectual disabilities. About 1 in 1,000 natural infections with measles causes *encephalitis,* an inflammation of the brain, which can result in lasting injury as well as deafness. About one to three in 1,000 who develop measles die from it. In very rare cases, years after an infection, it can cause something called subacute sclerosing panencephalitis (SSPE). It's an awful disease to see as there's no treatment for it, and it is almost always fatal (95 percent).

>> Mumps, also in the MMR vaccine, causes more serious symptoms as well. Mumps can cause meningitis (inflammation of the meninges surrounding the brain and spinal cord) in about one in seven infected. Most recover without a problem, but about one in 1,000 of those with meningitis develop encephalitis, which can be quite serious.

>> Rubella also can cause learning disabilities and deafness, particularly in those affected before birth or as infants.

For those who are autistic, it can be upsetting that parents say they would rather their children possibly die from measles or infect someone else who can die from measles than have their child be autistic. Autistic adults who live rich and enjoyable lives find this a bit distasteful. It's important not to let anyone be harmed by measles out of a fear of autism because this won't help anyone.

Myth: Vaccines contain harmful chemicals

Vaccines contain more than just antigens that create the antibodies that protect you from diseases. This shouldn't be a worry, though. Other ingredients are used to make sure those antigens reach us safely. These other ingredients (covered in Chapter 7) have been tested to ensure they aren't a cause for concern:

>> Preservatives keep the vaccine fresh (and include thimerosal, phenol, and 2-phenoxyethanol).

Thimerosal contains mercury. It's not the mercury found in fish, which is called methylmercury and can accumulate in our bodies. Instead, thimerosal breaks down into ethylmercury, which is water soluble, doesn't accumulate, and is easily flushed out. There's also another even more important reason parents don't need to worry about this in vaccines. Since 2001, every scheduled childhood vaccine comes in a formulation that is free of mercury. The only vaccine that might contain thimerosal is a multi-use vial of the flu vaccine; single-use vials are commonly used instead. Almost no vaccines have thimerosal; thimerosal is used in the manufacturing, but not in the final product, of one brand of one tetanus vaccine that adolescents and adults may take.

>> Adjuvants (like aluminum salts or squalene) strengthen the immune response.

>> Stabilizers (like gelatin) allow for vaccine transportation and storage.

>> Other ingredients may be used in vaccine production and removed once the vaccine is finished, but some traces can remain. These can include antibiotics (to prevent bacterial contamination, like neomycin), inactivating agents (to kill viruses and inactivate toxins, like formaldehyde), and materials used in cell cultures (egg proteins, cell lines).

Formaldehyde sounds like a chemical we don't want. It's used to inactivate viruses or toxins so they don't hurt you and is then removed. There can be trace amounts in some vaccines. This amount is so small that a newborn has 50 to 70 times the amount in the vaccine already in their body.

REMEMBER

The other ingredients are studied closely to make sure they don't cause any unexpected problems. If you do have an allergy to one of these, it's important to let your healthcare provider know. Antibiotics that commonly cause allergies are not included, but some people may have allergies to the antibiotics included. Gelatin, a common ingredient in food, can also be a cause of allergies.

Reviewing Vaccine Recalls

There are systems to catch mistakes if any are made. If the CDC, the FDA, the vaccine manufacturer, or other independent clinical studies identify a problem with a vaccine, these vaccines can be recalled.

Vaccine recalls are usually not because the vaccines are ineffective or unsafe. Recalls are usually done by companies voluntarily in case there may be an issue.

They usually occur because testing of some lots showed a possible problem, but not one that anyone has seen. For example:

>> A somewhat recent withdrawal occurred after a glass vial broke in production and there was concern that some of the vaccine bottles might have glass particles. No injuries or issues were ever seen.

>> Another recall was issued after testing showed bacteria had possibly grown in some vials, but after looking for any signs of infection in those who reported side effects, none were ever found.

There have been vaccines that have been suspended until there is more investigation. In the 1990s, use of the first rotavirus vaccine was suspended after some children had *intussusception*, where they had a bowel blockage after one part of their bowel slid past another. Although this was rare — and actually infections like rotavirus itself can cause this — the vaccine was suspended. Later versions of the rotavirus vaccine found it to be a rare adverse reaction to the vaccine — and actually more commonly brought about by other causes.

THE SWINE FLU VACCINE ROLLOUTS

In 2009, another pandemic was on the horizon — the swine flu or H1N1 influenza virus. This wasn't even the first time a potential swine flu epidemic caused worry and a rapid rollout of a vaccine.

In 1976, a type of swine flu swept through the army post Fort Dix in New Jersey, killing one soldier and sickening numerous others. Gerald Ford, the president at the time, determined that a national vaccination against the swine flu was necessary and promised to vaccinate every American.

Things didn't go well with this vaccine. The first doses weren't effective against the virus. Subsequent vaccines weren't effective in children. Then 94 people who had gotten the vaccine developed Guillain-Barré syndrome, which can cause temporary paralysis. And then the expected pandemic failed to arrive at all.

Fortunately, in 2009, we didn't see this. Because the production of flu vaccines is never immediate, there was not enough vaccine produced right away for everyone. The vaccine was distributed first to those most in need, including healthcare workers, pregnant women, small children, and those caregivers of small children. The H1N1 (swine flu) vaccine was then included as part of the regular flu vaccine in subsequent years. This flu type was included, in some form or another, in every year's seasonal vaccine over the next decade as it continued to circulate. The H1N1 in the vaccine is labeled as pdm09-like (pandemic 2009).

4

The Part of Tens

IN THIS PART . . .

Herald the vaccine pioneers.

Understand why some diseases have no vaccines.

Look back at pandemics throughout history.

Find tips for keeping your immune system working.

IN THIS CHAPTER

» Defeating smallpox

» Getting rid of rabies

» Overcoming polio with two different vaccines

» Meeting the man behind many modern vaccines

Chapter **12**

Five People Who Created Ten (Or More) Modern Vaccines

Rarely is one person responsible for the creation of a new vaccine. Scientists don't work in a vacuum, and it really does "take a village" to bring new ideas to fruition. However, a few men and women were the pioneering force behind certain vaccines and, in at least one case, the driving force behind a number of vaccines. This chapter covers five people responsible for at least ten modern vaccines.

Edward Jenner: Snuffing Out Smallpox

If you think about the history of vaccines at all — and it's okay if, like most people, you don't — the one name you may remember from the past was the man behind the first smallpox vaccine, Edward Jenner, an English physician. Jenner wasn't the first to try to eliminate smallpox, and he wasn't even the first to try inoculating with cowpox, a similar but harmless virus that often affected milkmaids. But he was the first to try to apply scientific methods and keep scientific data on his experiments.

Smallpox killed around 400,000 Europeans every year in the 1770s. Of those who survived, many were scarred. It caused a third of the cases of blindness in Europe. Prior to Jenner's work, a type of prevention called inoculation or variolation entailed scraping a small amount of fluid from a smallpox lesion into the skin. While this decreased the rate of deaths, it didn't eliminate them, as a certain number of people still developed severe cases of smallpox.

In 1796, Jenner took a small amount of matter from what was thought to be a cowpox lesion on the hand of a dairymaid and scraped it into the skin layers of an 8-year-old boy. The boy became mildly ill with cowpox. After he recovered, Jenner inoculated him with material from a smallpox lesion, and the boy didn't become ill, even after Jenner repeated the inoculation. Clearly, this wouldn't have been considered ethical today, but it did convince people that his method worked.

Jenner's method spread quickly, and the smallpox rate dropped. Jenner himself made little money off his discovery, but he did earn himself the lasting title of "The Father of Vaccination." Smallpox was declared completely eradicated from the world in 1979.

Louis Pasteur: Ridding the World of Rabies

Rabies wasn't a common disease in people; it was transmitted to humans only after they'd had contact with a rabid animal (usually after being bitten by a dog). However, because it was always fatal, it was a dreaded disease. Once symptoms were present, there was no stopping the progression.

Louis Pasteur, a French scientist, had been working on the transmission of rabies in animal species long before he tried his discoveries on a 9-year-old boy who'd been bitten 14 times by a rabid dog in 1885. Pasteur had discovered that the rabies virus became less virulent over time by using material from the dried spinal cords of rabid rabbits.

Because Pasteur wasn't a medical doctor but a scientist, he couldn't administer the material himself but had to call on medical friends to assist him. The material from the rabbits was injected into the boy's abdomen over 13 days, and he never developed rabies. Since the previous treatment for rabies bites was searing the bits with a red-hot iron, this was a major improvement, and Pasteur became well known for his vaccination against rabies.

TECHNICAL STUFF

Pasteur also worked on a vaccine for fowl cholera and on an anthrax vaccine to protect both sheep and cattle before he used his rabies vaccine on a human. He worked on fowl cholera (which is known now as *Pasteurella multocida*, a common cause of infection after cat and sometimes dog bites), and he realized that pathogens can be weakened over time, which can make vaccines less likely to cause the illness they were meant to prevent. This helped him develop an anthrax vaccine also made from live but weakened bacteria. This was the first live attenuated vaccine. Others would follow, including measles, mumps, rubella, and varicella. Rabies, though, is now only an inactivated vaccine in the United States.

Jonas Salk and Albert Sabin: Putting Polio Behind Us

The first documented polio outbreak in the United States occurred in Vermont in 1894. The outbreak resulted in 18 deaths and 132 cases of permanent paralysis. The actual poliovirus was isolated and identified in 1908. In 1916, an epidemic in New York City killed 2,000 people, and the summers, when most cases occurred, became a time for keeping children indoors and away from crowds.

Polio had been identified as a cause of paralysis, mostly but not only in children — President Franklin D. Roosevelt was probably its best-known victim, becoming paralyzed at age 39 in 1921. Rows and rows of iron lungs for children and adults took over hospitals. Most were confined to the "Iron Lung," which forced air in and out of the lungs, since breathing muscles were paralyzed in some polio patients. Most children spent two weeks in these boxes before they were able to breathe again on their own. While just 1 to 2 percent of people who contracted polio became paralyzed, with 98 percent having only mild symptoms, the outbreaks every few years still spurred a race for a vaccine.

In 1952, the number of polio cases in the United States surged, with 21,000 cases of paralysis. Summer outbreaks of polio once again frightened parents into keeping their children off the streets and away from crowds.

Some theorize that as sanitation improved, fewer infants contracted the polio virus at a young age, while they still carried some maternal antibodies. Because of maternal antibodies, their cases were generally mild, but the antibodies protected them from developing the disease again. With less exposure at a young age due to better sanitation, children were then more vulnerable as they got older and lost their maternal antibody protection, and they were more likely to develop the disease.

Jonas Salk didn't create the first polio vaccine; several polio vaccines preceded his but failed, either because they resulted in polio, because they resulted in allergic reactions, or because of their testing methods. But his vaccine, which protected against all three types of polioviruses, was the first to gain widespread use.

Salk's vaccine was an injectable killed virus, meaning that there was no chance, if properly produced, that people given the vaccine would get polio from it. After vaccination began in 1955, cases dropped from 45,000 per year to just 910 in 1962 in the United States. Today, the inactivated polio vaccine is the only one given in the United States. There has been no transmission of polio in the United States since 1979, and no wild-type polio has been brought by a traveler to the United States since 1993.

TECHNICAL STUFF

Like many scientists working with viruses and bacteria, Salk spent time working on an influenza virus while in school. In later life, he spent time trying to develop a vaccine against human immunodeficiency virus (HIV), a disease for which no vaccine yet exists.

At the time of Jonas Salk's vaccine, some scientists believed that live vaccines were still the most effective in preventing disease. Dr. Albert Sabin, an immigrant from Eastern Europe, developed a live polio vaccine that can be given orally in a syrup or on a sugar cube.

Because Salk's vaccine had suffered a setback after one manufacturer, Cutter Laboratories, incorrectly produced it, resulting in 40,000 cases of polio and 200 children with some degree of paralysis, Sabin's vaccine was more readily accepted and replaced Salk's vaccine for many years.

However, the live vaccine taken by mouth was, in rare cases, reactivated in the intestinal tract, causing between six and eight cases of paralysis per year in the late 1980s and 1990s. Because of this, a modified version of Salk's vaccine became the only polio vaccine used in the United States.

Sabin's vaccine, first used extensively in the late 1950s, is still used in many countries today, especially where its ease of use makes it a better choice than the inactive injectable Salk vaccine.

Maurice Hilleman: The Master of Modern Vaccines

Although few people outside the scientific community know his name, no one has had more influence on the current childhood vaccination lineup than microbiologist Maurice Hilleman. The number of vaccines he created (40) far exceeds the seven we need to reach a total of ten in this chapter, but the ones listed in this section are perhaps the best known.

Hilleman grew up as the eighth child, after his mother and his twin died in childbirth, on a farm in Montana during the Great Depression. He was a scientist rather than a medical doctor; he was the first to recognize that the sexually transmitted disease chlamydia was caused by bacteria rather than a virus and can be successfully treated with antibiotics.

Here are a few of the best-known vaccines that Hilleman created:

>> Hilleman developed his first vaccine, against Japanese encephalitis, in 1944, to save troops fighting in the Pacific from the disease.

>> Among Hilleman's live vaccines still used today are the measles, mumps, and rubella vaccines. He also combined the three vaccines, making it possible to protect against all three deadly diseases with just one injection. (See Chapter 6 for more on these vaccines.)

>> Hilleman was also the creator of the vaccines for varicella (chicken pox), *Haemophilus influenzae* bacteria, hepatitis A, hepatitis B, *Neisseria meningitidis*, and *Streptococcus pneumoniae*. (Check out Chapter 6 for details.)

Hilleman helped prevent an epidemic in the United States of the Hong Kong influenza outbreak in 1957, while working with Walter Reed Hospital. While 2 million died worldwide, only 70,000 died in the United States due to the 40 million vaccines given after being developed over a short four-month period. He was instrumental in the understanding of antigenic drift and shift in the influenza virus and the way it mutates each year, necessitating re-vaccination every year.

Hilleman's development of the mumps vaccine grew from his daughter Jeryl Lynn's case of the mumps. He took material from her swollen glands and used it to develop the mumps vaccine by weakening it. This mumps strain, the Jeryl Lynn strain (which actually included two variants often called by her initials, JL-1 [or JL-5] and JL-2), is still used in mumps vaccines today.

Hilleman considered his work on the hepatitis B vaccine one of his greatest achievements. His vaccine was later modified to be grown in yeast rather than treated blood serum, creating the first vaccine based on recombinant technology. The hepatitis B vaccine can prevent liver damage, including liver cancer, making it the first vaccine to protect against a type of cancer.

Like many pioneers, Hilleman was often impatient and brusque, especially when dealing with bureaucracies. But like him personally or not, it's impossible to deny the incredible effect he had on vaccine development.

Chapter **13**

Ten Diseases Without Vaccines, from A to Z

V accines have come a long, long way, but they haven't come all the way to curing every disease — not yet, anyway. Why are some diseases difficult if not impossible to create a vaccine for, and will this ever change in the future? The reasons why some diseases still flourish are many and complex. While some may be overcome in the next few decades, others may continue to elude researchers.

Some diseases are difficult to create vaccines for. Others do not have the financial incentive for companies to invest in. Worries about regulations and lawsuits may limit others. There have been initiatives like the Coalition for Epidemic Preparedness Innovations, working with the World Health Organization, nonprofits, and other governments to support research and development for important diseases that have not had vaccines. The rapid development of vaccines for COVID-19 shows that with the right motivation and funding, there may be answers to some of the tougher vaccine questions.

This chapter covers ten diseases without vaccines at the time of writing.

Avian Influenzas (Bird Flu)

Birds can infect people with type A influenza viruses that normally affect only bird species, including domestic poultry such as chickens, ducks, or turkeys. Fortunately, these viruses rarely jump to people from birds, but when they do, they can cause serious illness, including pneumonia or even death.

Because many variations of type A influenza viruses infect primarily birds, it's hard to develop a vaccine that prevents all of them. In the United States, a vaccine has been created, but against only one specific type of bird flu, H5N1. This vaccine is stockpiled and not in general use for the American public.

TECHNICAL STUFF

Bird flu can cause low pathogenic avian influenza, or LPAI, or highly pathogenic avian influenza, or HPAI. These designations refer to the degree of illness in birds, not people. LPAI may cause only very mild symptoms in birds. HPAI, on the other hand, can cause serious or even fatal illnesses in birds. Both LPAI and HPAI can cause serious illness in people.

Bird flu in people causes symptoms similar to other flus, such as fatigue, fever, headache, muscle aches, runny or stuffy nose, reddened eyes, and mild upper respiratory symptoms such as a cough. However, cases of H5N1 viruses in China, Africa, and the Middle East have caused severe pneumonia, with a 50 percent death rate. There are also serious infections and deaths due to H7N9. H7N7 has been responsible for illness and one human death (in a veterinarian), and H7N3 has been known only to cause mild illness in poultry workers.

Fortunately, bird flus generally don't jump from birds to people, although the potential is there. This is usually more of a problem for poultry farms, as many birds can get sick. Care while handling farmed as well as wild birds or fowl can help prevent cases of bird flu. Also fortunately, bird flu has only rarely been transmitted from one person to another. Antiviral medications can help treat bird flu if it develops. See Chapter 2 for an introduction to type A influenza viruses.

Cytomegalovirus (CMV)

There's a good chance — up to 85 or 90 percent — that you've had cytomegalovirus, or CMV, at some point in your life if you're an adult. A third of children under age five have already had the virus. CMV spreads through contact with bodily fluids, such as blood, breast milk, saliva, semen, urine, and even tears. Transplanted organs can also carry the virus. CMV often causes only mild symptoms, usually flu-like symptoms such as fever, fatigue, headache, and muscle aches. Sounds like nothing to worry about, and for most people, it isn't.

However, CMV, like the virus that causes shingles, the varicella virus, remains in a dormant state in your body and can cause major health issues if your immune system becomes weakened. If a pregnant woman who has never had CMV catches it during pregnancy, she has a 40 percent chance of passing it on to her unborn baby, who can have lifelong health issues from the virus. Pregnant women who have already had CMV can also transmit the virus via the placenta, although the risk of transmission is less than 1 percent.

WARNING

Babies exposed to CMV before birth can be born prematurely or have a low birth weight. Some women miscarry or suffer stillbirth. Of those born with CMV, 90 percent will have no symptoms at birth. Of those who do have symptoms, 10 percent may die soon after birth. Of those with symptoms, many have hearing loss; some have seizures, developmental delays, an enlarged spleen, or liver damage. Some are born with a rash, smaller than normal head size, jaundice, or eye damage to the retina. Of the majority with no symptoms at birth, some may be found to have hearing loss, but three out of four will have no long-term health problems.

Organ transplant patients or other people who have a decreased immune response, as well as those who are in intensive care without known immune system issues, may experience a reactivation of CMV. Reactivation of the virus can sometimes cause specific symptoms in persons with different types of immunosuppression: damage to the retina of the eye (particularly in advanced AIDS), severe gastrointestinal issues, life-threatening pneumonia (particularly in lung transplants), or infection of the brain *(encephalitis)*. In people who have had an organ transplant, CMV can also cause rejection of the new organ. Antiviral medications can help prevent the complications of CMV after organ transplant or in people with severely compromised immune systems, such as those with AIDS (covered later in this chapter).

Although congenital CMV affects around twice as many infants as Down syndrome, many people aren't aware of the virus's potential for long-term harm in susceptible populations. Lack of public awareness and demand for a vaccine have slowed the research and development of a vaccine for CMV. However, clinical trials have made progress as new technologies for vaccines have been developed.

Epstein-Barr Virus (EBV)

Epstein-Barr virus (EBV), a human herpes virus called HHV4, like many other viruses, often affects people in childhood. Around 50 percent of children under age five have already had it in the United States, and most have mild cases with only minor viral symptoms. The virus spreads easily through contact with infected bodily fluids, including saliva.

EBV causes 90 percent of cases of a more familiarly named illness due to its transfer through saliva — mononucleosis, also sometimes called "kissing disease." Mononucleosis affects one to two million Americans each year. Most common in teens and college students between the ages of 15 and 24, mononucleosis causes fever, body aches, swollen lymph nodes, fatigue, headaches, loss of appetite, nausea, rash, sore throat, and vomiting. The sore throat can be severe.

Symptoms, particularly fatigue, can last for weeks or even months. EBV can sometimes cause more serious symptoms, such as a ruptured spleen, an enlarged liver, or other liver-related side effects such as jaundice.

WARNING

EBV can also contribute to development of certain cancers, particularly gastric or nasopharyngeal cancers of the epithelial cells, the cells that make up the lining of body surfaces, and B cell cancers such as Burkitt's and Hodgkin's lymphomas. B cells are part of your body's immune system. Worldwide, EBV-related cancers affect around 200,000 people and kill 140,000 every year.

EBV infection might also trigger autoimmune conditions, and this is being studied.

Scientists have been working on a vaccine for EBV, but as of yet, no clinical trial has shown to be effective enough to bring a vaccine into production.

Hepatitis C

Hepatitis C infects around 1.75 million people worldwide every year. Approximately 2.4 million Americans have the disease. Over half the people initially infected with hepatitis C develop chronic disease. Like hepatitis A and B (covered in Chapter 6), this virus can have serious effects on the liver. Unlike hepatitis A and B, no vaccine yet exists for hepatitis C. Other than their effects on the liver, the three similarly named viruses aren't related.

Hepatitis C spreads mostly through contact with blood. Mother-baby transmission during pregnancy and transmission during sex, particularly in gay men, are also possible. Most cases occur through shared needles in IV drug users. Blood transfusions, needlesticks, non-sterile tattoos, or poorly sterilized medical equipment can also transmit the disease. Blood products in the United States are checked for hepatitis C.

Hepatitis C is the main cause of cirrhosis of the liver that progresses to the point of needing a liver transplant. Between 5 and 25 percent of chronic hepatitis C patients develop cirrhosis within 10 to 20 years; those who develop cirrhosis have a 1 to 4 percent chance each year of developing liver cancer.

Most people who are infected with hepatitis C experience no initial symptoms. Those who are symptomatic may experience abdominal pain, dark urine, fatigue, loss of appetite, nausea, or vomiting. Yellowing of the white of the eyes and jaundice can also occur. Those who are symptomatic with initial infection are the most likely to clear the virus on their own.

There are several reasons why a hepatitis C vaccine hasn't been developed yet:

>> There are at least seven different genotypes and over 60 subtypes of hepatitis C; developing a vaccine against all types is difficult.

>> Animal testing is also complicated by the fact that the only animals that are affected by the virus are chimpanzees; these animals are expensive, and there are also ethical concerns to using them for experimental testing.

>> Surface antigens (aka "Wanted" photos) are difficult to produce.

>> It's more complicated to design an efficacy trial.

>> New treatments may have dampened the interest in a vaccine. There may be less financial incentive.

Fortunately, medications can cure many hepatitis C infections. Different antiviral treatments work against different genotypes, and treatment can take several months.

Herpes Simplex Virus (HSV) 1 and 2

The herpes simplex viruses 1 and 2 cause different types of disease. Neither can be prevented by vaccine, although scientists are working on it. Both forms hang around in latent form in your body for life; outbreaks occur at intervals. Having one form of the virus doesn't protect you against getting the other.

Between 50 and 80 percent of Americans have HSV 1, the virus that causes cold sores on the lips, also called fever blisters. Around one in six between the ages of 14 and 49 have HSV 2, which causes genital herpes. You can be infected with type 1 through oral contact, including oral sex. However, HSV 1 can cause both oral and genital or anal lesions. Type 2 is passed through genital contact. Most of the time, both types are asymptomatic but can still be transmitted to another person.

WARNING

Cold sores are initially painful and annoying, with burning and tingling in the area, but otherwise harmless. They often occur in response to stress. Genital herpes, however, can have serious side effects for an unborn baby if a pregnant woman carries genital HSV. If you have active genital herpes, your healthcare provider may recommend a Cesarean section rather than a vaginal delivery.

Neonatal herpes infection affects one in 5,000 to 7,500 infants. Signs of infection usually occur within the first month of life and can have widespread effects, from central nervous system effects, including seizures, to organ or eye damage.

Immunocompromised people such as transplant recipients, cancer patients, and people with HIV who have HSV 1 can have serious side effects such as encephalitis (infection of the brain) or eye infection.

Antiviral medications can treat outbreaks, but they're not a cure. A vaccine that prevents HSV infections hasn't yet come onto the market, although potential vaccines are under investigation.

HIV/AIDS

The virus that causes HIV, human immunodeficiency virus, which weakens the immune system and is passed through bodily secretions, probably originated in chimpanzees and jumped to humans in the late 1800s and early 1900s, spreading in Kinshasa, the Democratic Republic of Congo, in the 1920s.

HIV in the United States was first recognized in 1981 when five gay men in Los Angeles developed a rare lung infection called *Pneumocystis carinii* pneumonia. Around the same time, an outbreak of an unusual cancer called Kaposi's sarcoma occurred in New York City and California in gay men. Because the immune deficiency disorder that led to both conditions appeared to be sexually transmitted and to affect gay men, it was originally called gay-related immune deficiency (GRID).

During the 1980s, cases of what was now called AIDS, or acquired immune deficiency syndrome, were diagnosed all over the world. Women who had sex with infected men had been infected, as well as newborn or breastfeeding children whose moms had the infection. Hemophiliacs were especially affected as the virus made its way into the blood supply. Intravenous drug users were also at high risk.

Symptoms of primary infection with HIV are similar to other viruses; the disease is very contagious at this initial stage. The infection will then become chronic, but you take antiviral medications to treat it and prevent further progression. If untreated, the chronic infection can progress to AIDS.

REMEMBER

Antiretroviral treatments have significantly decreased deaths from AIDS. Treatment is started as soon as possible to avoid any progression of the illness. A person with HIV on antiretrovirals can live just as long as someone without HIV. PrEP (pre-exposure prophylaxis), taken daily, and PEP (post-exposure prophylaxis), taken daily for one month after exposure, have proved very effective in preventing HIV infection in high-risk populations.

Although the infection and death rates have dropped significantly, HIV still poses a serious health issue. AIDS is still the leading cause of death worldwide for women of childbearing age. Rates of HIV remain high in some parts of the world. In some countries in southern Africa, close to one in five are infected. There and throughout the world, HIV programs have enrolled many in treatment. The goal is to have 90-90-90 (90 percent of those infected are tested and know their diagnosis, 90 percent of those who know their diagnosis are on treatment, 90 percent on treatment have viral load suppression). Most of the countries in southern Africa have either met these targets or are close, though COVID-19 has led to some setbacks in HIV programming. Treatment, though, is not a cure. A vaccine would change this tremendously.

While a vaccine against HIV hasn't yet been developed, some scientists continue to work on developing one. It has been complicated scientifically. Early trials have not been successful. We are still learning from patients whose immune systems are able to control HIV and remain disease free, with an undetectable virus.

Lyme Disease

With warm weather comes ticks. If you live in a tick-infested state, you have probably heard of Lyme disease, a tick-borne illness that can cause long-lasting symptoms in some people.

Lyme, Connecticut, has the dubious distinction of being the first place this illness was first recognized in the United States. In 1976, a group of parents in three close-by towns noticed their children had developed swollen joints, especially knees. Some also had nonspecific symptoms such as fever, headaches, muscle aches, and weakness. A total of 39 children and 12 adults developed these symptoms over summer and fall. Of these, 25 percent also had an unusual bull's-eye rash before the joint symptoms began.

Two types of bacteria, *Borrelia burgdorferi* and *Borrelia mayonii*, cause Lyme disease in the United States. Deer ticks and black-legged ticks carry the bacteria, passing it on to humans they bite. Because these ticks are so small, you may not notice that you've been bitten. The tick must attach for at least 36 to 48 hours to transmit the bacteria to you. Larger ticks, such as dog ticks, don't carry the bacteria that causes Lyme disease.

Avoiding ticks by staying out of wooded areas, using approved insect repellents, wearing long sleeves, and wearing light-colored clothing to make ticks easier to see can help avoid a tick bite. A thorough check for ticks after spending time outside is also beneficial.

A tick bite initially leaves a small bump or reddened area. This doesn't mean that you have Lyme disease. The typical Lyme bull's-eye rash — alternating bands of red and white — occurs three to 30 days after exposure, growing slowly to as much as 12 inches. The bull's-eye rash can also appear in areas far from the original bite. At least 25 percent of people with Lyme never have the rash. Left untreated, a person with Lyme may develop joint pain, neurological problems, severe fatigue, heart issues, or liver inflammation.

Blood testing for Lyme disease looks for antibodies to the bacteria that cause Lyme disease. A positive test doesn't always indicate a current infection; you may have developed antibodies from a past mild infection. If this test, called the ELISA test, is positive, it's followed by more specific testing called a Western Blot test.

Antibiotics, usually doxycycline or amoxicillin, treat Lyme disease effectively if given early. Sometimes a longer treatment time of several weeks becomes necessary.

Around 476,000 people are diagnosed and treated for Lyme disease each year in the United States, although not all may actually have had the disease. The CDC reports just 30,000 diagnosed infections per year, still a fairly large number. But with such large numbers of presumptive cases, why hasn't a vaccine been created yet? The answer is that there was a Lyme vaccine, LYMErix. It was approved in 1998 by the United States Food and Drug Administration (FDA), but it was withdrawn from the market in 2002.

The vaccine was almost 80 percent effective, which was good news. It wasn't tested or available for children, though, and they often have the most tick exposures. The vaccine then had a lot of publicity in the media, with lots of reports of side effects, though without studies to determine cause. It was not clear whether the joint pains some experienced, but which weren't more common than in the general population, were related to the vaccine.

The vaccine also came out around the time that the vaccine for rotavirus, a diarrheal illness in children, was being withdrawn from the market for complications in infants. So there was even more attention on the vaccine.

A watchdog group filed class action suits against the Lyme vaccine, citing long-term complications from it, although the FDA was unable to verify the claims. However, with sales falling, negative media publicity, and suits pending, the manufacturer withdrew the vaccine from the market.

Currently, dogs can receive a Lyme vaccine, and several companies have vaccines in early clinical trials for humans.

Respiratory Syncytial Virus (RSV)

Respiratory syncytial virus, more commonly known as RSV, affects nearly all children by their second birthday. Many have mild symptoms. However, between 75,000 and 125,000 children, most under a year old, end up hospitalized with the virus every year in the United States for pneumonia or inflammation of the small airways in the lungs.

Worldwide, between 66,000 and 234,000 infants die each year from RSV, most in developing countries. RSV also affects elderly adults; between 14,000 and 62,000 each year are hospitalized in the United States.

The reason that there's no vaccine for RSV isn't for lack of trying. However, a huge setback for an RSV vaccine occurred in the 1960s, when an inactivated vaccine in clinical trials allowed for a more virulent form of lower respiratory tract disease, called enhanced RSV disease, to develop in RSV-vaccinated children. A large number were hospitalized, and two infants died.

After this terrible experience, attention turned to live vaccines only for RSV. More recently, subunit vaccines, based on a protein section of the virus, have also been considered. Currently, around 60 potential vaccines for RSV are in developmental or preclinical development, with a smaller number in clinical trial development.

Problems with development of an RSV vaccine include the following issues:

>> RSV most commonly has severe effects in young infants. The maternal antibodies a young infant is born with can interfere with the baby's development of antibodies against RSV.

>> Animal models and subjects for developmental trials are hard to find, as well as expensive.

>> RSV viruses are diverse, divided into types A and B and then even further subdivided into different genotypes and variants. Finding one vaccine that works against all forms of RSV is difficult.

West Nile Virus

West Nile virus first appeared in the United States in 1999. But its origins go back to the West Nile area in Uganda, where it made an appearance in 1937. The virus is carried from infected birds to mosquitoes that bite them, and then to humans bitten by mosquitoes carrying the virus. Mosquitoes carrying the virus, *Culex* species mosquitoes, have been found in every state except Alaska and Hawaii.

REMEMBER

Not all mosquitoes carry the virus, so every bite isn't a reason to run to the doctor. Even if cases of West Nile virus have occurred in your area, very few mosquitoes carry the virus. The type of mosquito that carries the virus — yes, there are actually different types of mosquitoes — is most active at dawn and dusk. However, if you show symptoms, call your healthcare provider immediately.

Most people infected by West Nile virus have no symptoms at all. But around 20 percent develop West Nile fever, with flu-like symptoms besides fever including body aches, headache, fatigue, nausea, vomiting, or rash.

Fewer than 1 percent develop serious neurological effects such as meningitis or encephalitis. Symptoms can include confusion, headache, stiff neck, high fever, seizures, muscle weakness, or partial paralysis. Some side effects, such as muscle weakness, can be permanent. The elderly are most likely to be affected by serious infection, which in some cases is fatal.

Although vaccines are in clinical trials for humans, none have yet been marketed or approved by the FDA. Cost effectiveness may be an issue in developing a vaccine, and figuring out where the next West Nile outbreak may occur can also be difficult. A vaccine for horses, which are also affected by West Nile, has been approved, but the regulations for veterinary vaccines are less stringent than those for people.

REMEMBER

The best way to avoid West Nile Virus is to wear long-sleeved clothing and use an approved insect repellent any time you're out and about where you're likely to be bitten, such as wooded or grassy areas. Remove any sources of standing water to eliminate places for mosquitoes to breed. Wearing mosquito nets over your head may be overkill, but if you're a really cautious type, or if you spend lots of time in mosquito-infested areas, it may be a good idea.

West Nile virus can't be caught from another person. Blood products can carry the infection; in the United States, blood products used for transfusion are screened for the virus.

Zika Virus

Zika is another disease transmitted by mosquitoes. Zika was also first found in Uganda. The first large recorded outbreak in 2007 in Micronesia was followed by outbreaks in 2013 and 2015. More than 1 million cases were reported in 2016 worldwide. While the incidence of Zika virus has declined since the last big outbreak in the Americas in 2016 — including a few cases in the United States, most travel-based — the virus still exists. Another outbreak can occur at any time.

Zika virus is transmitted by the *Aedes* species mosquito, which bites both day and night, mostly in the early morning and late afternoon or early evening. The virus can also be sexually transmitted or transmitted during pregnancy from mother to baby. Blood products can also carry the infection.

WARNING

The potential effects of Zika virus on unborn babies whose moms contract it during the first three months of pregnancy are especially severe. Babies born after contracting the virus in utero may have very small heads, called *microcephaly*, and other birth defects. Some babies die in utero, are born prematurely, or are stillborn. Zika virus can lead to learning disability and lifelong disabilities for these babies.

Like West Nile and other viruses, around 80 percent of people infected with Zika virus have no symptoms at all. Symptoms that can occur are common to many other illnesses and include headache, fever, lack of energy, muscle soreness, nausea, rash, or red eyes (conjunctivitis). Symptoms usually last between two and seven days.

A small percentage of infected people can develop Guillain-Barré syndrome, with paralysis, muscle weakness, or neurological issues. Severe symptoms occur most frequently in children and older adults.

Currently, no vaccine for Zika virus exists, although many have been or are still in clinical trials. Because the outbreaks appear to have decreased, less sense of urgency to develop a vaccine exists. Ethical challenges, such as the difficulties in testing a vaccine on pregnant women, also affect the ability to create a vaccine.

Chapter **14**

The Ten Most Lethal Major Pandemics

The COVID-19 pandemic, while obviously fresh in our minds, is far from the first or worst world pandemic, and it certainly won't be the last. Fortunately, today there's a vaccine to protect against the disease, which hasn't been the case throughout history, when countries around the world were decimated by various pandemics.

REMEMBER

By definition, a *pandemic* affects the whole world, while *epidemics*, although sometimes just as lethal, affect only certain areas.

In this chapter, we take a look back through history at some of the worst pandemics ever documented and their effects on the world, both in the long and short term. While the numbers of some of the major pandemics may not seem that high, keep in mind that the world's population was much smaller 2,000 years ago, and the percentage of the population that died much higher.

Antonine Plague (165–180)

Increased trade routes with parts of the globe previously unreached can have mixed blessings. So the Romans found when the silk and spice trade with the East increased, bringing with it not only highly prized goods but an illness not seen in Rome before.

Called the Antonine Plague, after the ruling family of the time, or the Plague of Galen, after the Greek physician, the pandemic was possibly caused by smallpox. But we don't know for sure. It caused fever, diarrhea, sore throat, and skin sores. Those who got sick either got better in two weeks or did not. Without knowing more and without any testing, we can't be sure what caused it. Some have even thought it might have been caused by measles, influenza, or even a relative of Ebola.

It lasted for 15 years, spread from one end of the Roman empire to the other, and caused the deaths of 60 to 70 million people, between 25 and 33 percent of the population. At the disease's height in Rome, nine years after it first began, between 2,000 and 5,000 people died every day from the illness.

The well-trained Roman army took a tremendous hit. Because of the loss of men to the plague, new recruits — less well trained, not always committed to their new tasks — had to be taken in to fill the ranks. This allowed the Germanic army to cross the Danube River into Roman territory for the first time.

During the same time period as the Antonine Plague, outbreaks of a similar disease were occurring in the Near East, affecting the Han empire. Quite possibly it was the same disease.

Plague of Justinian (541–750)

Also known as the Justinian or Justianic plague, this outbreak occurred in the mid-500s and continued in waves for two centuries. Named for the emperor of the Byzantine (Eastern Rome) Empire, Justinian, the plague was caused by the same bacteria, although possibly a different strain, that caused the later and larger outbreak in the 1300s.

The Justinian plague, which began in Egypt and spread north and east from there, may have killed as many as 25 to 50 million people, or 25 percent of the population. While the Eastern Roman Empire was most affected, cases may have occurred, according to anecdotal information, as far away as England.

As with later plague outbreaks, transportation of grain on ships and supply transports spread the bacteria, as these brought rats, although person-to-person spread also contributed. Fleas and vermin were the main source of infection.

The Justinian plague finally vanished in 750 CE, although the plague would definitely return. While the plague may have contributed to the downfall of the Eastern Roman Empire, scholars today don't believe it was the main cause.

Bubonic Plague (Black Death) (1346–1353)

When the word "plague" comes up (hopefully not too often in daily conversation), this is the plague that probably comes to mind. The plague shown in movies with solemn men swinging lanterns and intoning "Bring out your dead." The plague that supposedly inspired the children's song "Ring Around the Rosie." The lyrics described the rash (a ring of roses) that sufferers developed, the posies of herbs used for protection or to block the stench, sneezing (*a-tishoo*), followed by a whimsical but grim "We all fall down."

While the plague of the mid-1300s was one of the most deadly, plague outbreaks occurred regularly in pockets of the known world. Possibly originating in China, the 1346 plague hopped a ride to Europe and Africa, generally thought to have spread via fleas that lived on the rats that infested sailing ships. It's possible that human lice also carried the bacteria *Yersinia pestis* from person to person.

Between 75 and 200 million people died in the plague outbreak, which added up to between 17 and 45 percent of the known world's population. This was before travel became more extensive and frequent. Christopher Columbus hadn't yet sailed the ocean blue and found the New World after discovering the world wasn't flat.

The mortality rate was 90 percent if you caught the disease. There are different ways a plague can present, depending in part on transmission: bubonic, septicemic, and pneumonic. This plague is associated with bubonic disease (with buboes or painful swelling). However, there would have been septicemic plague cases, which can develop from untreated bubonic plague or directly from flea bites. Person-to-person transmission through droplets can spread pneumonic plague, or it can develop from untreated bubonic and septicemic plague. Today, with treatment, the mortality rate from the bubonic and septicemic plague is 10 percent, but the pneumonic plague remains very deadly. The pneumonic form of disease is almost always fatal if not treated within the first 24 hours with the appropriate antibiotics, which only came about in the 1900s.

Cholera (1846–1860)

Like many more recent pandemics, the cholera pandemic of 1846 spread via transport. The increased ability to travel from one part of the globe to another, while beneficial in many ways, has proven to be a two-edged sword in others.

Cholera outbreaks still plague areas of the world with insufficient sanitation and contaminated water. But at different times in history, outbreaks have circled the globe to become pandemics. The third and most deadly such pandemic began in India in 1846 and continued until 1860.

Vibrio cholerae, the gram negative bacteria that causes cholera, largely spreads via fecal-oral transmission, especially through stool-contaminated food and water. Cholera, once introduced, can persist in water and even accumulate in seafood, like oysters. While 80 percent of people infected have few symptoms, 20 percent develop severe vomiting and diarrhea, which can lead to dehydration and death within a few hours if not treated with rehydration.

British soldiers carried cholera from India to other outposts, and from there the bacteria spread via rivers and other waterways. By 1848, cholera infected Europe, and from there it was carried to seaports in the United States. Irish immigrants, leaving Ireland due to the potato famine, also helped spread the disease to North America. Water shipped to the inner parts of the country helped spread the bacteria. By the early 1850s, cholera had reached the Far East, where local outbreaks continued for years. Around this time, cholera was finally realized to be waterborne, as John Snow mapped cases of cholera and tied them to one Broad Street water pump. Before that, the disease was often thought to be due to miasmas or bad air and blamed on poor living conditions and sometimes religion.

Approximately 1 million people died in Russia alone during the 1846 cholera pandemic. Because the pandemic continued over a number of years and caused numerous small outbreaks, it's difficult to say how many people died altogether, but England alone experienced outbreaks that killed tens of thousands.

REMEMBER

Clean water standards and a better knowledge of sanitation has helped keep cholera at bay, but outbreaks still regularly do occur where there are fewer resources for sanitation and drinking water. The largest recorded number of cases occurred in Yemen, with an epidemic beginning in 2016 that has affected over 2.5 million people, resulting in close to 4,000 deaths. Another outbreak spread in Haiti in 2010 after the bacteria was introduced there, resulting in about 10,000 deaths.

Third Plague Pandemic (1855–1960)

The last plague pandemic began in 1855 and was considered active with outbreaks continuing through 1960. Once cases fell to less than 200 per year, the World Health Organization (WHO) declared the pandemic over. Although it occurred over a long time period, the fact that it killed between 12 and 15 million people during that time still makes it a deadly pandemic.

This plague pandemic, like the 1346 one covered earlier in this chapter, started in China and traveled on ships to points around the world. However, unlike earlier plague pandemics, this one caused far more deaths in certain parts of the world than it did in others. Most of the deaths occurred in China, India, and Indonesia, along with British and French colonies. But the death tolls in Great Britain, the United States, and Central and South America were quite low.

REMEMBER

The idea that germs caused illness and that scientists from different countries, working together, can eradicate a common enemy began with the third plague. The public health initiatives begun during this plague helped keep death rates down in the areas where they were used and set a precedent for international cooperation during worldwide pandemics.

The bacteria that cause the plague still exist in the rodent population, especially prairie dogs, in the Southwestern United States, with around seven new cases occurring each year. Outbreaks still occur every few years in Madagascar, with just over 200 dying in 2017.

Influenza (Russian Flu) (1889–1890)

You've never heard of the Russian flu, which started in — surprise — Russia and circled the globe in just four months? Because it's been somewhat overshadowed by the death rate of the 1918 flu, most people outside of infectious disease experts haven't heard of it. But the Russian flu was the first pandemic outbreak to spread throughout a world connected by faster and newer modes of travel, such as railways.

The Russian flu was originally thought to have been possibly caused by the H3N8 or H2N2 virus. However, some researchers today theorize that what was thought to be the flu may actually have been a coronavirus because of the large number of nervous system effects reported. (See Chapter 3 for more about the coronavirus.)

The fatality rate from the Russian flu was similar to the later 1957 and 1968 flu pandemics — around 0.15 percent. This was much less than the 1918 pandemic death rates of around 10 times higher. The R0, or the number of people infected by each person, was figured to be around 2, similar also to the 1957 and 1968 flu pandemics, as well as the 1918 pandemic (see the next section).

Once the virus reached the East Coast of the United States, it was easily spread throughout the country via the railways. At first downplayed by public health officials and newspapers, the flu began to be taken more seriously as the death toll rose. The death toll in the United States reached 13,000 cases out of a total population of 60 million. Worldwide, the death toll was around 1 million people and the world had one-fifth the population we do now. Relatively, this would be much greater than the current COVID-19 outbreak.

Influenza (Spanish Flu) (1918–1919)

When it comes to influenza outbreaks, nothing so far compares to the 1918 influenza pandemic commonly called the Spanish flu. Killing around 50 million people worldwide, the Spanish flu — an H1N1 influenza A virus that probably began as a bird flu — infected around one-third of everyone on earth. The mortality rate was around 10 percent, and many of the victims were adults between the ages of 20 and 40. Around 675,000 Americans died during the pandemic.

TECHNICAL STUFF

Despite its name, the Spanish flu didn't originate in Spain. Because Europe was still fighting World War I at the time of the outbreak, most countries severely restricted their news reporting. Spain, being neutral, was putting out the most reports of the growing flu outbreak, which made it seem as though most cases started or came from there.

The Spanish flu came in three waves during 1918–1919. While the first wave wasn't much more virulent than other flu outbreaks, the second wave — a mutated version — was much more deadly, capable of killing a previously healthy person seemingly overnight. Lung damage was severe in many people, which medical personnel today surmise came from an immune overreaction called a cytokine explosion. There also could be superinfections with bacteria, which there weren't yet antibiotics for.

The war contributed to the rapid spread of the virus, as troops carried it from one continent to another. Maintaining production of materials needed for the war made putting quarantines into place difficult. The third wave of the virus proved just as deadly as the second.

The flu that spread in 1918 never entirely went away. The virus mutated and spread to different animals. The virus became a regular old flu and continues to spread year to year every flu season.

Influenza (Asian Flu) (1957–1958)

Like the 1918 pandemic discussed in the preceding section, the influenza pandemic of 1957 — sometimes called the Asian flu — was a type A influenza virus that probably originated as a bird flu. The virus, an H2N2 subtype, started in East Asia in February 1957 and reached the United States by the summer of the same year. Between 1 million and 4 million people died around the world, with between 70,000 and 116,000 dying from the flu in the United States. Around 25 percent of the U.S. population contracted the virus.

The Asian flu was a new type of virus, one that hadn't been seen before. Few people carried any immunity to the virus, which increased the death rate. One deadly aspect of this flu was its ability to cause life-threatening pneumonia even without any superimposed bacterial infection.

The fatality rate was less than 1 percent — somewhere between 0.2 and 0.6 percent — compared to the death rate from most flus of less than 0.1 percent. Rapid development of a vaccine slowed the spread of the virus, which faded by 1958, although outbreaks continued for the next ten years.

Human Immunodeficiency Virus (HIV) (1981–Present)

You may not consider human immunodeficiency virus (HIV) to be a plague unless you were alive in the 1980s and saw how it appeared seemingly out of nowhere. It affected only certain groups of people, with no real explanation of what caused it. The viral cause was isolated two years after the disease first appeared in 1981, but the virus had already infected people on five continents.

As a bodily fluid–borne infection, HIV can be passed through sex, especially spreading among men who have sex with men; spread via sharing needles; or transmitted from mother to baby in utero or during breastfeeding. HIV is not transmitted through saliva or tears.

Today, HIV has spread around the world, infecting around 65 million people, with 25 million dying from the disease. In some countries, most people who are infected are women, as transmission of the virus occurs most commonly during heterosexual sex. Countries test blood supplies for the virus; some also distribute clean needles to intravenous drug users. But 1.7 million new infections were diagnosed in 2019 worldwide, and 38 million people were living with HIV.

Antiviral treatments have extended the lives of millions of people with HIV, although treatments still don't reach everyone, particularly in low- to middle-income countries. The worldwide goal is to achieve 90–90–90, whereby 90 percent of those infected are tested and know their diagnosis, 90 percent who know they are infected are on treatment, and 90 percent on treatment are suppressed with an undetectable viral load. Treatment is prevention, as those who have an undetectable viral load do not transmit the infection to others.

COVID-19 (2020–Present)

For many people, the year 2020 began with fear. A new illness was affecting China, and news pictures of people being chased through the streets or locked into their houses did nothing to decrease fears. It seemed that a new plague had threatened China and, soon enough, the rest of the world as well.

The new virus eventually acquired a name — COVID-19, a type of coronavirus caused by SARS-CoV-2. Symptoms included respiratory issues as well as fever, fatigue, and muscle aches. In March, the World Health Organization declared COVID-19 a pandemic. Statistics were difficult to pin down at first, but eventually it became evident that the virus was much more deadly than influenza, especially among certain populations. Around 3 million people have died of COVID-19, including nearly 600,000 in the United States, at this point.

REMEMBER

Lockdowns, mask regulations, and shutting down of schools and businesses were all part of the fabric of life in 2020 and into 2021 around the world. So much is still unknown about what will happen in the next few years due to COVID-19.

REMEMBER

Vaccine programs will certainly have an impact, although these work only if a large number of people are vaccinated worldwide. If vaccination programs aren't able to vaccinate enough people and COVID-19 is allowed to continue to spread, it's not certain how long vaccine immunity will last and whether mutations will lead to booster shots. Vaccine hesitancy exists in the United States and elsewhere as people question the vaccine's safety, although millions have been vaccinated safely and the risk of COVID-19 outweighs any vaccine side effects.

Chapter **15**

Ten Ways to Boost Your Immune System

Vaccines are the best way to ward off potentially dangerous illnesses. But you can also take steps every day to make yourself less susceptible to illness, boosting your immune system, and making you better able to resist all kinds of bugs. Many of the changes you can make won't cost you anything and, as a bonus, will make you feel better every day of your life.

Getting Your Vaccinations

REMEMBER

If you wander through the array of supplements that promise to boost your immune system at the pharmacy, you may find it hard to believe that getting vaccinated is the best immune system booster of all. But it's true: The best protection against diseases that used to be commonplace is getting vaccinated. While you can't be vaccinated against every disease, you can be vaccinated against many. For diseases that don't have a vaccine yet, consider the rest of the suggestions in this chapter.

Decreasing Stress

Yes, stress can affect your immune system and make you more susceptible to getting sick. So how can you suffer from less stress when life is so stressful? The way you react to stressors — and everyone has them — can affect the way your immune system reacts.

WARNING

Some people go through life chronically angry — at everything. A car that pulls out in front of them, a long line at the grocery store, a perceived snub from a co-worker — everything generates a stress response. While it might seem like getting angry, yelling, and "getting it out of your system" would be a good thing, it really isn't. Staying in a continual "flight or fight" state triggers the release of chemicals such as cortisol that, over time, put a lot of stress on your immune system. In the short run, cortisol is beneficial, but if your levels are chronically high, you can produce fewer lymphocytes, white blood cells that help you fight off illnesses.

Learning to manage stress can take time and effort. Techniques that teach you to calm your breathing and certain types of exercise such as yoga, meditation, or prayer can help you get through stressful situations while keeping stress from becoming chronic.

Eating Well

Micronutrients such as vitamins and minerals as well as macronutrients — protein, carbs, and fats — all help you maintain a healthy immune system. But your food, not the local health food store, is the best way to get the nutrients you need. Supplements can't overcome a poor diet, and too many supplements over-promise on their benefits.

Everyone has days where their diet falls off the nutritionally sound chart. Your goal should be to eat well most of the time. What does it mean to eat well?

» First off, get enough protein. Protein is the building block for cells, and falling short can have serious side effects. Beef, fish, poultry, eggs, tofu, cheese, and nuts all supply protein.

» You need carbohydrates too — but the right kind, in the right amounts. Complex carbohydrates, like vegetables, beans, and whole grains, are good — a bag of chips, not so much. Refined sugars in large amounts can cause harm to many parts of your body, including your immune system.

>> And although fat has become a bad word in dietary terms, good fats are another essential part of healthy eating. Nuts, olive oil, fatty fish, and even dark chocolate can help boost your immune system.

REMEMBER

Eating well, with an adequate amount of fruits and vegetables along with protein and good fats, will supply the nutrients you need and, in most cases, eliminate the need for supplements.

REMEMBER

If you have nutritional deficiencies, taking dietary supplements can help. It is unlikely that you are missing any vitamins in your diet. Megadoses of certain supplements, such as zinc, can actually harm rather than help your immune system. Always talk to your healthcare provider before taking supplements of any kind in large amounts. We discuss supplements in more detail later in this chapter.

Maintaining a Healthy Weight

WARNING

Maintaining a healthy weight goes hand in hand with eating well (see the preceding section). Both overweight and underweight individuals can have immune system disruptions:

>> Excess weight can cause inflammation, which affects your immune responses in a number of ways, including by decreasing your white blood cell function and making you more susceptible to infection, as we have seen with COVID-19 and influenza.

>> Being underweight, particularly if you have a protein deficiency, can also affect your immune response, as seen with tuberculosis.

Keeping your weight within a normal range can help keep not only your immune system but all your major organs functioning well.

Getting Enough Sleep

"To sleep, perchance to dream," as Shakespeare said. Sleep is another area where falling short can have negative effects on your immune system. Too many things keep us from sleeping well and sleeping long enough and deeply enough to get into sleep states necessary for good health.

Disturbed or shortened sleep periods can cause inflammation and increased hormone stress levels. This can also disrupt some of our coordinated immune system responses. Some studies showed that restricted sleep can also decrease antibody production after vaccination.

WARNING

Taking sleeping pills every night can make sleep issues worse in the long run, so try to limit their use. Adults need seven to eight hours of sleep a night.

Exercising for Immunity

Exercise in moderation to keep your immune system humming. But "moderation" can be hard to define — does a stroll around the block count? Ten minutes on the exercise bike or treadmill? Five hours a day lifting weights at the gym?

Walking half an hour a day, fast enough to get your heart rate up; bicycling; or working out at the gym three or four times a week can reduce your stress levels, which in turn can help your immune system. Regular exercise can also increase the way antibodies and white blood cells circulate through your body. Exercise can also help you control your weight, which in turn has benefits for your immune system.

REMEMBER

Getting 150 minutes per week of moderate exercise, or 75 minutes of strenuous exercise, can pay big dividends toward boosting your immune system and making your feel better at the same time.

Saying No to Smoking

Smoking has an array of negative effects on your entire body, including your immune system. The numerous chemicals in tobacco, not just nicotine, can increase inflammation, particularly in your lungs, making you more susceptible to infection and tissue destruction. Smoking also has negative effects on your immune system's ability to respond to infection by decreasing white blood cell activity.

In some people, smoking can increase the risk of autoimmune diseases such as rheumatoid arthritis or multiple sclerosis. Smoking can cause a harmful overactive immune response that leads to these conditions and can lead to persistent chronic inflammation. Inflammation can lead to increased tissue destruction and more negative effects on cells that help keep your immune system in balance.

One of the best things you can do for your immune system? Quit smoking — or don't ever start.

Drinking Only in Moderation

You may have heard that a glass of red wine a day can help keep you healthy. There's some truth in this; antioxidants in red wine may have a positive benefit on your immune system, but only in moderation. And "moderation" may be far less alcohol than you think: Experts recommend no more than one drink per day for women and two for men.

But the downside of alcohol consumption is that drinking to excess does a lot of harm to your immune system. Any more than that can disrupt your immune system, starting in your gastrointestinal tract after your first swallow. Alcohol decreases the number of healthy microbes in your GI tract, damages immune cells that line the intestine, and interferes with your body's healing processes.

Staying Connected

Although it isn't yet clearly understood, and it may sound a little out there, there seems to be a definite connection between your mental state and your immune system. You've probably heard that "Happiness is a state of mind" or "You're only as happy as you make up your mind to be." While life circumstances can certainly steal joy from all of us, staying involved with life no matter what the circumstances may affect your immune system as well as your outlook.

Of course this isn't easy, or always possible. But some studies have shown a definite link between people's attitudes and involvement with other people and their immune system's functioning. So don't pooh-pooh the benefits of staying active, connected, and involved on your physical as well as your mental health.

Don't have family around? Look for other people to befriend or to get involved with. Develop hobbies that you can share with others. Volunteer somewhere. Talk to your neighbors when you're out walking. There's no reason to live a lonely, isolated life unless you're a person who really cherishes solitude. You don't have to be social every minute of the day, but maintain relationships that make you happy. Work on relationships that don't. And hopefully, your immune system will reward your efforts.

Considering Supplements

Okay, maybe all the tips earlier in this chapter sound like too much work. Why can't you just go to the health food store, pick up a few bottles of multivitamins, probiotics, and other heralded immune boosters, and call it good? While some supplements may have an effect on your immune system, most really don't. Others haven't been tested in any meaningful way — as in a well-designed clinical trial in humans, not small animals — in the amounts normally found in supplements. And the amounts used in the studies often exceed what's found in the average supplement.

REMEMBER

However, if you want to add supplements to other methods of getting your immune system humming, there are a few you can try. Again, make sure to run anything you're taking past your healthcare provider:

» **Vitamin D** deficiency is much more common than once thought. We spend less time outside, and sun exposure manufactures vitamin D in the skin. Those who have lower vitamin D levels are more at risk for respiratory infections, but unfortunately supplementing vitamin D doesn't always reduce infections. Because vitamin D is a fat-soluble vitamin, excess amounts are stored in the body and can be harmful, so check any supplements with your doctor. Be careful, as too much vitamin D can be dangerous.

» **Vitamin C** is often thought to help the immune system fight off infections. Fruits such as oranges, tangerines, and strawberries and veggies such as spinach and kale supply you with vitamin C. Unfortunately, it won't necessarily keep the cold at bay. If you eat a balanced diet, you should have enough vitamin C. Talk to your doctor if you think it might help you.

» **Zinc,** when taken in proper quantities, helps boost immune cell development. Zinc deficiencies occur most commonly in the elderly, affecting as many as 30 percent, due to poor dietary intake or medications that decrease zinc absorption, such as diuretics. Talk to your doctor if you think you need more zinc in your diet.

» **Vitamin B6** also plays a role in keeping your immune system working well. Beef, chicken, fish, and fortified cereal help meet your daily needs. Talk to your doctor if you think you might be deficient.

Index

A

abscesses, 38
acellular vaccines
   defined, 58
   pertussis and, 88
acetaminophen, 139
achy muscles, as side effect, 115
acquired immunodeficiency syndrome (AIDS), 204–205
adenoviruses
   cancer and, 39
   colds and, 35
   in COVID-19 vaccine, 51
adjuvants
   allergic reactions to, 166–167
   defined, 10–11
   as vaccine ingredients, 106–108
adult vaccines
   catching up on missed childhood vaccines, 160
   COVID-19, 149–150
   diphtheria, 150–151, 155
   herpes zoster, 151–153
   influenza, 148–149, 153–155
   pertussis, 150–151, 155
   pneumococcus, 99–100, 156
   during pregnancy, 156–157
   shingles, 151–153
   Tdap, 150–151, 155
   tetanus, 150–151, 155
   whooping cough, 150–151, 155
adverse reactions, 116–120
   allergic reactions
      avoiding, 117
      ingredients, 165–170
      overview, 16
   anaphylactic reactions
      avoiding, 117–118
      COVID-19, 170
      overview, 16
   antibiotics
      C diff, 65
      superinfections, 38
   avoiding, 117–118
   body aches, 115
   causes of, 106–110
   COVID-19 vaccine, 52–53, 170–171
   fainting, 116
   fatigue, 115
   febrile seizures, 118–119
   fever, 114–115
   gastrointestinal issues, 115
   Guillain-Barré syndrome, 119
   headaches, 115
   herpes zoster vaccine, 152
   Hib vaccine, 89
   hives, 112
   hospitalization and, 116
   immune response, 114–116
   injection pain, 111–112
   itching, 112
   lightheadedness, 116
   myths regarding, 180–181
   overview, 16
   rashes, 112–113
   redness, 113
   reporting, 116–117
   rheumatic fever, 38
   skin reactions, 111–114
   swelling, 113–114
   thrombocytopenia, 120
   wheal, 111
AIDS (acquired immunodeficiency syndrome), 204–205
alcohol, immune system and, 223
allergic reactions, 165–170
   to adjuvants, 166–167
   to antibiotics, 165–166
   avoiding, 117
   immune response vs., 169
   overview, 16
   to preservatives, 166–167
   to stabilizers, 166–167
   types of, 168–169
   to vaccine ingredients, 165–168

Almeida, June, 32
aluminum, 108
American Academy of Family Physicians, 144
American Academy of Pediatrics, 144
anaphylactic reactions. *See also* adverse reactions;
    allergic reactions
    avoiding, 117–118
    COVID-19 vaccine, 170
    overview, 16
anthrax
    overview, 60
    vaccines for, 82
antibiotics
    allergic reactions to, 165–166
    hospitalization and, 65
    for Lyme disease, 206
    preventing bacteria in vaccines, 11
    side effects from
        C diff, 65
        rashes, 113
        superinfections, 38
    as vaccine ingredients, 110
    vaccines vs., 64–66
antibodies
    COVID-19 test for, 47
    exercise and, 222
    IgE, 168
    IgM, 125
    overview, 10
    passive immunity, 126
antigens
    antigenic drift, 19–20
    bacteria and, 58
    children and, 184
    hemagglutinin, 93
    historical decrease in usage of, 127
    overview, 10, 106
    testing for, 47
    as vaccine ingredients, 107
antiretrovirals
    AIDS and, 204
    defined, 25
anti-vaxxers, 176–179
Antonine Plague, 212
Asian flu pandemic (influenza pandemic of 1957), 217
aspirin

    taking after vaccination, 139
    taking before injection, 115
AstraZeneca vaccine, 51–52
autism, 187–188
avian flus
    overview, 20
    pandemics, 200, 216–217

B

Bacillus anthracis, 60
bacteria
    anthrax
        overview, 60
        vaccine for, 82
    antibiotics vs. vaccines, 64–66
    attenuated, 71
    Bacillus anthracis, 60
    Bordetella, 62
    Borrelia burgdorferi, 206
    Borrelia mayonii, 206
    Campylobacter jejuni, 119
    cholera
        overview, 60–61
        pandemics, 214
        Pasteur and, 194–195
        vaccine delivery method, 160
    Clostridium difficile, 65
    Clostridium tetani, 63, 87
    Corynebacterium diphtheriae, 61, 87
    diphtheria
        overview, 61, 131
        vaccines for, 86–87, 113, 131–132, 142–143,
            150–151, 155
    Hib
        overview, 62
        vaccines for, 88–89, 132
    Lyme disease, 205–207
    meningococcus
        overview, 62
        travel and, 159
        vaccines for, 97–98, 142
    Mycobacterium bovis, 186
    Mycobacterium tuberculosis, 63
    Neisseria meningitidis, 62, 97
    overview, 58–59

Pasteurella multocida, 194

pertussis
  overview, 62, 131
  vaccines for, 88, 131–132, 142–143, 150–151, 155

pneumococcus
  overview, 62
  vaccines for, 98–101, 156

Salmonella Typhi, 64

Streptococcus pneumoniae, 62, 98–100

tetanus
  overview, 63, 131
  vaccines for, 87, 113, 131–132, 142–143, 150–151, 155

toxins, 11–14, 59

tuberculosis, 63–64

typhoid
  overview, 64
  travel and, 159

Vibrio cholerae, 60, 214

viruses vs., 11–14, 57–58

Yersinia pestis, 213

baculoviruses, 93

bird flus
  overview, 20
  pandemics, 200, 216–217

Black Death (bubonic plague), 213

blood clots, 52–53

body weight, immune system and, 221

boosting immune system, 219–224

Bordetella, 62

Borrelia burgdorferi, 206

Borrelia mayonii, 206

breastfeeding, 126

bubonic plague (Black Death), 213

Burkitt's lymphoma, 202

C

C Diff (*Clostridium difficile*), 65

Campylobacter jejuni, 119

cancer
  colds as potential cure for, 39
  COVID-19 and, 163
  influenza and, 163
  mononucleosis and, 202
  vaccines and, 162–163

CDC (Centers for Disease Control and Prevention)
  boosters, 150–151
  COVID-19, 48
  Lyme disease, 206
  pneumococcal vaccines, 99
  reporting side effects to, 180–181
  shingles vaccine, 103
  travel, 158
  vaccine schedules, 144
  website for, 56

cellulitis, 113

childhood vaccines
  antigens and, 184
  catching up on, 144–146
  diphtheria, 131–132, 142–143
  helping children through, 135–136
  hepatitis A, 140
  hepatitis B, 128–129
  Hib, 132
  HPV, 141–142
  importance of, 127
  influenza, 133–134
  IPV, 132–133
  laws, 140–141
  measles, 137
  MenACWY, 142
  mumps, 137
  myths regarding, 181–184
  overview, 125
  passive immunity, 125–126
  PCV13, 134
  pertussis, 131–132, 142–143
  pneumococcus, 100–101
  rotavirus, 129–130
  rubella, 138
  Tdap, 131–132, 142–143
  tetanus, 131–132, 142–143
  varicella, 139–140
  whooping cough, 131–132, 142–143

cholera
  overview, 60–61
  pandemics, 214
  Pasteur and, 194–195
  travel and, 160

cirrhosis, 202
clades, 94
clinical trial phases, 76–77
Clostridium difficile (C Diff), 65
Clostridium tetani, 63, 87
CMV (cytomegalovirus), 200–201
cold chain, 13
cold sores, 203
colds, 34–40
  causes of, 34–35
  defined, 34
  differentiating from other
    illnesses, 35–40
  as potential cure for cancer, 39
Common Cold Unit, 32
community effectiveness, 78–79
conjugate vaccines, 73, 98
coronaviruses
  causes of, 34–35
  COVID-19
    cancer and, 163
    coping with, 56
    detecting infection, 46–49
    herd immunity, 53–55
    long, 46
    overview, 14–15
    pandemic, 42–44, 218
    protecting against, 55–56
    risks for hospitalization, 45–46
    symptoms, 44–45
    testing for, 47
    vaccination after infection, 173
    vaccine ingredients, 171–172
    vaccine reactions, 170–173
    vaccines for, 50–53, 149–150
    variants of, 48–49
  defined, 34
  identifying, 32–33
  MERS, 41–42
  RSV
    overview, 207
    symptoms, 35–36
  SARS, 40–41
  symptoms, 35–40
Corynebacterium diphtheriae, 61, 87
costs of vaccines, 75–76

COVID-19
  cancer and, 163
  coping with, 56
  detecting infection, 46–49
  herd immunity, 53–55
  long, 46
  overview, 14–15
  pandemic
    overview, 218
    start of, 42–44
  protecting against, 55–56
  risks for hospitalization, 45–46
  symptoms, 44–45
  testing for, 47
  vaccines for
    adults, 149–150
    ingredients in, 171–172
    overview, 50–53
    reactions to, 170–173
    vaccination after infection, 173
  variants, 48–49
coxsackieviruses, 35
Cutter Incident, 182–183
cVDPV (vaccine derived polio virus), 183
cytokine explosion, 216
cytomegalovirus (CMV), 200–201

D

dehydration, 101
delivery methods for vaccines, 110–111
deoxyribonucleic acid (DNA), 18
dermatone, 27
diabetes, 65
diet, immune system and, 220–221
diphtheria
  overview, 61, 131
  vaccines for
    adults, 150–151, 155
    children, 131–132, 142–143
    effectiveness, 86–87
    rashes, 113
DNA (deoxyribonucleic acid), 18
double-blind studies, 77
drift (antigenic drift), 19–20
dry stage of Ebola, 28

E

Ebola, 27–29
EBV (Epstein-Barr virus), 201–202
efficacy of vaccines, 78–80
eggs
  allergy to, 167
  growing viruses in, 11
  as vaccine ingredient, 110
Emergency Use Authorization, 77
encephalitis
  CMV and, 201
  defined, 86
  measles and, 137, 188
  vaccines for, 197
enteroviruses
  colds, 35
  polio, 22–23
epidemics. *See also names of specific illnesses*
  defined, 43, 211
  Ebola, 28
  H1N1, 21, 190
  MERS, 33
  SARS, 33
EpiPens (epinephrine pens), 118
Epstein-Barr virus (EBV), 201–202
erythema multiforme, 113
ethylmercury, 109
exercise, immune system and, 222

F

fainting, 116
fatigue, 115
FDA (Food and Drug Administration)
  ingredients approved by, 13
  Lyme disease, 206
  new vaccines, 74–75
  side effects, 116–117, 180–181
febrile seizures
  after vaccination, 118–119
  measles and, 137
fevers, 114–115
FLUAD/FLUZONE vaccine, 155
flus. *See also names of specific flus*
  bird flus, 20, 200
  cancer and, 163

colds vs., 36
coping with, 56
overview, 18–22
pandemics, 215–217
swine flu, 21, 190
vaccines for
  adults, 148–149, 153–155
  children, 133–134
  effectiveness, 93–95
  history of, 82
  yearly, 15
variants, 82
fontanelle, 98
Food and Drug Administration (FDA)
  ingredients approved by, 13
  Lyme disease, 206
  new vaccines, 74–75
  side effects, 116–117, 180–181
Ford, Gerald, 190
formaldehyde, 110, 189
fungi, 12

G

Gardisil 9 vaccine, 92
gastrointestinal issues, as side effect, 115
gay-related immune deficiency (GRID), 204
GBS (Guillain-Barré syndrome)
  overview, 119
  swine flu vaccine and, 168, 190
  Zika virus and, 209
gelatin, 109, 166
GRID (gay-related immune
      deficiency), 204
Guillain-Barré syndrome (GBS)
  overview, 119
  swine flu vaccine and, 168, 190
  Zika virus and, 209

H

H (hemagglutinin) proteins, 20
Haemophilus influenzae type b (Hib)
  overview, 62
  vaccines for
    children, 132
    overview, 88–89

Hamre, Dorothy, 32

headaches, as side effect, 115

hemagglutinin (H) proteins, 20

hemagglutinin antigen, 93

hepatitis
 A, 140
 B, 128–129
 C, 202–203
 vaccines for, 89–91

herd immunity
 defined, 8
 overview, 53–55
 R0 and, 79–80

herpes simplex virus (HSV), 203–204

herpes zoster
 overview, 27
 vaccines for
  adults, 151–153
  overview, 102–104

hesitancy toward vaccines,
 176–179

Hib (Haemophilus influenzae type b)
 overview, 62
 vaccines for
  children, 132
  overview, 88–89

Hilleman, Maurice, 196–197

history of vaccines, 80–83

HIV (human immunodeficiency virus)
 antiretroviral treatment,
  204–205
 overview, 24–25
 pandemic, 217–218

hives, as side effect, 112

Hodgkin's lymphoma, 202

hospitalization
 allergic reactions, 165
 antibiotics, 65
 chicken pox, 86
 COVID-19, 45–46
 influenza, 153
 rotavirus, 129
 RSV, 207
 vaccination side effects, 116

HPV (human papillomavirus)
 overview, 92
 vaccines for, 141–143

HSV (herpes simplex virus), 203–204

human immunodeficiency virus (HIV)
 antiretroviral treatment, 204–205
 overview, 24–25
 pandemic, 217–218

human metapnuemoviruses, 35

human papillomavirus (HPV)
 overview, 92
 vaccines for, 141–143

I

ibuprofen, 139

idiopathic thrombocytopenic purpura (ITP), 169

IgE (immunoglobulin E) antibody, 168

IgM antibodies, 125

immune system, 114–116
 alcohol and, 223
 allergic reactions vs. response from, 169
 antigens and, 10
 cytokine explosion, 216
 diet and, 220–221
 disorders, 163–164
 exercise and, 222
 myths regarding, 184
 sleep and, 221–222
 smoking and, 222–223
 socializing and, 223
 stress and, 220
 supplements and, 224
 vaccines and, 120–121, 219
 weight and, 221

immunity
 herd immunity
  defined, 8
  overview, 53–55
  R0, 79–80
 natural
  myth regarding, 186–187
  overview, 10
 passive, 125–126
 vaccines and, 16

Immunization Action Coalition, 140

immunoglobulin E (IgE) antibody, 168

inactivated vaccines
 overview, 72
 polio, 132–133

IND (Investigational New Drug), 75
infections
  colds, 34–40
  COVID-19
    detecting, 46–49
    vaccination after, 173
  noroviruses, 24–25
influenzas. *See also names of specific influenzas*
  bird flus, 20, 200
  cancer and, 163
  colds vs., 36
  coping with, 56
  overview, 18–22
  pandemics, 215–217
  swine flu, 21, 190
  vaccines for
    adults, 148–149, 153–155
    children, 133–134
    effectiveness, 93–95
    history of, 82
    yearly, 15
  variants, 82
ingredients
  2-phenoxyethanol, 109
  adjuvants
    allergic reactions, 166–167
    defined, 10–11
    overview, 106–108
  aluminum, 108
  antibiotics, 110
  antigens, 107
    antigenic drift, 19–20
    bacteria and, 58
    children and, 184
    hemagglutinin, 93
    historical decrease in usage of, 127
    overview, 10, 106
    testing for, 47
  COVID-19 vaccine, 171–172
  eggs
    allergic reaction, 167
    preventing bacteria in, 11
    proteins, 110
  formaldehyde, 110, 189
  gelatin, 109, 166
  latex, 117, 167–168

in Moderna vaccine, 172
myths regarding, 188–189
in Pfizer vaccine, 171–172
phenol, 109
preservatives
  allergic reaction, 108
  overview, 11, 106
  as vaccine ingredient, 166–167
production materials
  defined, 11
  overview, 106
  types of, 110
stabilizers
  defined, 11
  overview, 106, 109
  as vaccine ingredient, 166–167
testing, 13
thimerosal, 108–109
in vaccines, 10–11
yeast, 167
injections
  anaphylactic reactions and, 110
  chicken pox, 113
  children, 135–136
  COVID-19, 171–172
  DTaP, 131
  EpiPen, 168
  febrile seizures and, 96
  hepatitis
    children, 140
    pregnancy, 129
    vaccine for, 90–92
  Hib and
    children, 132
    importance of, 89
  HIV and, 25
  influenza
    adults, 149
    vaccine for, 133
  mRNA vaccines, 50
  pain in site of, 111–112
  PCV13, 134
  pneumococcus, 99
  rabies, 159
  shingles

injections *(continued)*
    adults, 152
    overview, 103
   smallpox, 104
   subcutaneous and subdermal, 111
   tetanus, 65
Institutional Review Board, 75
intramuscular delivery method, 111
intranasal delivery method, 111
intussusception
   in children, 130
   defined, 102
   hesitancy toward vaccines and, 190
Investigational New Drug (IND), 75
itching, as side effect, 112
ITP (idiopathic thrombocytopenic purpura), 169

J

Japanese encephalitis, 197
Jenner, Edward
   overview, 193–194
   smallpox, 81
   variolation, 178
Johnson & Johnson vaccine
   anaphylactic reactions, 170
   ingredients in, 172
   as viral vector vaccine, 51–52

L

Lancet, The, 187–188
latex allergies, 117, 167–168
laws on vaccinations
   children, 140–141
   hesitancy toward vaccines and, 179
lightheadedness, as side effect, 116
live pathogen vaccines
   immune disorders and, 164
   overview, 70–72
long COVID-19, 46
lots, 13
Lyme disease, 205–207
Lynn, Jeryl, 95, 197

M

malaria, 160
measles
   encephalitis and, 188
   overview, 25–26, 95
   vaccines for
      children, 137
      effectiveness, 95–97
      hesitancy toward, 177
      history of, 82–83
      rashes, 113
MenACWY vaccine
   overview, 98
   for teenagers, 143
meningococcus
   overview, 62
   vaccines for
      children, 97–98
      MenACWY, 142–143
mercury
   hesitancy toward vaccines and, 189
   thimerosal and, 109
MERS (Middle East respiratory syndrome)
   origin of, 33
   overview, 41–42
messenger RNA (mRNA) vaccines
   COVID-19 vaccine, 14, 171
   defined, 74
   overview, 50–52
metapnuemoviruses, 35
methylmercury
   hesitancy toward vaccines and, 189
   overview, 109
Middle East respiratory syndrome (MERS)
   origin of, 33
   overview, 41–42
MiraLAX, 52
Moderna vaccine
   anaphylactic reactions, 170
   emergency use authorization of, 51
   ingredients in, 172
molecular tests, 47
mononucleosis, 202

Montagu, Mary, 80
mosquitoes, 208–209
mRNA (messenger RNA) vaccines
  COVID-19 vaccine, 14, 171
  defined, 74
  overview, 50–52
mumps
  overview, 95
  vaccines for
    children, 137
    effectiveness, 95–97
    history of, 82–83
    rashes, 113
mutations, 18–20
Mycobacterium bovis, 186
Mycobacterium tuberculosis, 63

N

N (neuraminidase) proteins, 20
National Conference of State Legislatures, 141
National Institutes of Health, 75
National Vaccine Injury Compensation Program
  overview, 116
  website for, 183
natural immunity
  myth regarding, 186–187
  vaccinations vs., 10
Neisseria meningitidis, 62, 97
neuraminidase (N) proteins, 20
neurotoxicity, 108
noroviruses, 23–24
nucleic acid vaccines, 74

O

Onesimus, 80
oral delivery method, 111
orchitis, 95
Oxford vaccine, 51–52

P

pandemics. *See also names of specific illnesses*
  Antonine Plague, 212
  Asian flu, 217
  Bubonic Plague, 213

cholera, 214
COVID-19, 42–44, 218
defined, 43, 211
H1N1, 21, 190
HIV, 217–218
MERS, 33
Plague of Justinian, 212–213
Russian flu, 215–216
Spanish flu, 216–217
Third Plague Pandemic, 215
parainfluenza, 35
parasites, 12
passive immunity, 125–126
Pasteur, Louis, 194–195
Pasteurella multocida, 194
pathogens. *See also names of specific pathogens*
  adenoviruses
    cancer and, 39
    COVID-19, 51
    symptoms, 35
  anthrax
    overview, 60
    vaccine for, 82
  antibiotics vs. vaccines, 64–66
  attenuated, 71
  Bacillus anthracis, 60
  bacteria
    overview, 11–14
    viruses vs., 57–58
  baculovirus, 93
  Bordetella, 62
  Borrelia burgdorferi, 206
  Borrelia mayonii, 206
  Campylobacter jejuni, 119
  cholera
    overview, 60–61
    pandemics, 214
    Pasteur and, 194–195
    vaccine delivery method, 160
  Clostridium difficile, 65
  Clostridium tetani, 63, 87
  Corynebacterium diphtheriae, 61, 87
  coxsackieviruses, 35
  cytomegalovirus, 200–201
  defined, 8, 17

pathogens *(continued)*
  diphtheria
    overview, 61, 131
    vaccines for, 86–87, 113, 131–132, 142–143,
      150–151, 155
  Ebola, 27–29
  EBV, 201–202
  enteroviruses
    overview, 22–23
    symptoms, 35
  hepatitis
    A, 140
    B, 128–129
    C, 202–203
    vaccines for, 89–91
  Hib
    overview, 62
    vaccines for, 88–89, 132
  HIV, 24–25, 204–205
  HPV, 143
  HSV, 203–204
  influenzas
    bird flus, 20, 200
    cancer and, 163
    colds vs., 36
    coping with, 56
    overview, 18–22
    pandemics, 215–217
    swine flu, 21, 190
    vaccines for, 15, 82, 93–95, 133–134, 148–149,
      153–155
    variants, 82
  Lyme disease, 205–207
  measles
    overview, 25–26
    vaccines for, 82–83, 95–97, 113, 137
  meningococcus
    overview, 62
    travel and, 159
    vaccines for, 97–98, 142
  metapnuemoviruses, 35
  Mycobacterium bovis, 186
  Mycobacterium tuberculosis, 63
  Neisseria meningitidis, 62, 97
  noroviruses, 23–24

  overview, 11–12, 18, 59–64
  parainfluenza, 35
  Pasteurella multocida, 194
  pertussis
    overview, 62, 131
    vaccines for, 88, 131–132, 142–143, 150–151, 155
  pneumococcus
    overview, 62
    vaccines for, 98–101, 156
  Pneumocystis carinii, 204
  protection against, 58–59
  rhinoviruses
    overview, 22–23
    symptoms, 35
  rotavirus
    in children, 129–130
    overview, 101–102
  RSV
    overview, 207
    symptoms, 35–36
  Salmonella Typhi, 64
  smallpox, 29
  Streptococcus pneumoniae, 62, 98–100
  tetanus
    overview, 63, 131
    vaccines for, 87, 113, 131–132, 142–143, 150–151, 155
  toxins
    from bacteria, 59
    overview, 11–14
  tuberculosis, 63–64
  typhoid
    overview, 64
    travel and, 159
  vaccinia, 185
  varicella
    overview, 26–27
    vaccines for, 83, 85–86, 113, 139–140
  variola, 29
  Vibrio cholerae, 60, 214
  viruses
    bacteria vs., 57–58
    overview, 11–14
  West Nile virus, 208
  Yersinia pestis, 213
  Zika virus, 209

PCR (polymerase chain reaction), 47
PCV13, 134
PEG (polyethylene glycol)
  anaphylactic reactions and, 171
  in mRNA vaccines, 52
pertussis
  overview, 62, 131
  vaccines for
    adults, 150–151, 155
    children, 131–132, 142–143
    effectiveness, 88
Pfeiffer, Richard, 81
Pfizer vaccine
  anaphylactic reactions, 170
  emergency use authorization of, 51
  ingredients in, 171–172
phases, of clinical trials, 76–77
phenol, 109
PHN (postherpetic neuralgia), 151–152
Plague of Galen, 212
Plague of Justinian, 212–213
pneumococcus
  overview, 62
  vaccines for
    adults, 99–100, 156
    effectiveness, 98–101
Pneumocystis carinii, 204
polio
  overview, 23
  vaccines for
    history of, 82, 182
    inventors, 195–196
    polio, 132–133
polyethylene glycol (PEG)
  anaphylactic reactions and, 171
  in mRNA vaccines, 52
polymerase chain reaction (PCR), 47
polysaccharide vaccines, 59, 73
post-exposure prophylaxis
  AIDS and, 204–205
  overview, 25
postherpetic neuralgia (PHN), 151–152
precautions before vaccination, 169–170
pre-exposure prophylaxis

AIDS and, 204–205
  overview, 25
pregnancy
  cytomegalovirus and, 201
  HIV and, 25
  passive immunity, 126
  rubella and, 138
  vaccination during
    chicken pox, 86
    influenza, 95
    live vaccines, 71
    overview, 156–157
  Zika virus and, 209
preservatives
  allergies to, 166–167
  overview, 11, 106, 108–109
prions, 12
production materials
  overview, 11, 106
  types of, 110
prolines, 51
proteins
  from eggs, 110
  on influenza virus, 20
  naming flu vaccines, 94
  overview, 50–51
  vaccines with, 73
pseudomembranes
  defined, 61
  diphtheria, 86–87

R

R0
  herd immunity, 79–80
  overview, 53–54
  Russian flu, 216
  for varicella, 85
rabies
  overview, 194–195
  travel and, 159
randomized controlled trials, 76–77
rapid tests, 47
rashes, as side effect, 112–113

reactions, 116–120
  allergic reactions
    avoiding, 117
    ingredients, 165–170
    overview, 16
  anaphylactic reactions
    avoiding, 117–118
    COVID-19, 170
    overview, 16
  antibiotics
    C diff, 65
    superinfections, 38
  body aches, 115
  causes of, 106–110
  COVID-19, 52–53
  fainting, 116
  fatigue, 115
  febrile seizures, 118–119
  fever, 114–115
  gastrointestinal issues, 115
  Guillain-Barré syndrome, 119
  headaches, 115
  herpes zoster vaccine, 152
  Hib vaccine, 89
  hives, 112
  hospitalization and, 116
  immune response, 114–116
  injection pain, 111–112
  itching, 112
  lightheadedness, 116
  myths regarding, 180–181
  overview, 16
  rashes, 112–113
  redness, 113
  reporting, 116–117
  rheumatic fever, 38
  skin reactions, 111–114
  swelling, 113–114
  thrombocytopenia, 120
  wheal, 111
reactogenic vaccines
  defined, 52
  shingles and, 103
  side effects, 114

redness, as side effect, 113
reporting side effects, 116–117
respiratory syncytial virus (RSV)
  overview, 207
  symptoms, 35–36
Reye's syndrome, 115
rhinoviruses
  overview, 22–23
  symptoms, 35
ribonucleic acid (RNA), 18
risks for hospitalization, 45–46
Roosevelt, Franklin D., 132, 195
rotavirus
  in children, 129–130
  overview, 101–102
RSV (respiratory syncytial virus), 35–36, 207
rubella
  overview, 96
  pregnancy and, 138
  vaccines for
    children, 138
    effectiveness, 95–97
    history of, 82–83
    rashes, 113
Russian flu pandemic, 215–216

S

Sabin, Albert, 82, 133, 195–196
Salk, Jonas, 82, 133, 195–196
Salmonella Typhi, 64
SARS (severe acute respiratory syndrome)
  origin of, 33
  overview, 40–41
scheduling vaccines
  catching up on childhood vaccines, 144–146
  importance of, 15–16
sepsis, 98
septicemia, 98
severe acute respiratory syndrome (SARS)
  origin of, 33
  overview, 40–41
shift, 19–20

shingles
  overview, 27
  vaccines for
    adults, 151–153
    overview, 102–104
Shingrix, 103
side effects
  adverse reactions, 116–120
  allergic reactions
    avoiding, 117
    ingredients, 165–170
    overview, 16
  anaphylactic reactions
    avoiding, 117–118
    COVID-19, 170
    overview, 16
  antibiotics
    C diff, 65
    superinfections, 38
  body aches, 115
  causes of, 106–110
  COVID-19, 52–53
  fainting, 116
  fatigue, 115
  febrile seizures, 118–119
  fevers, 114–115
  gastrointestinal issues, 115
  Guillain-Barré syndrome, 119
  headaches, 115
  herpes zoster vaccine, 152
  Hib vaccine, 89
  hives, 112
  hospitalization and, 116
  immune response, 114–116
  injection pain, 111–112
  itching, 112
  lightheadedness, 116
  myths regarding, 180–181
  overview, 16
  rashes, 112–113
  redness, 113
  reporting, 116–117
  rheumatic fever, 38
  skin reactions, 111–114
  swelling, 113–114
  thrombocytopenia, 120
  wheal, 111
SIDS (Sudden Infant Death Syndrome), 119
sinusitis, 38
skin reactions, as side effect,
    111–114
sleep, immune system and, 221–222
smallpox
  eradicating, 104
  overview, 29
  vaccines for, 80–81, 193–194
smoking, immune system and, 222–223
Snow, John, 214
socializing
  immune system and, 223
  social distancing, 55
Spanish flu pandemic, 216–217
SSPE (subacute sclerosing panencephalitis), 188
stabilizers
  allergy to, 166–167
  overview, 11, 106, 109
Stevens-Johnson syndrome, 113
strep throat, 37–38
Streptococcus pneumoniae, 62, 98–100
stress, immune system and, 220
subacute sclerosing panencephalitis (SSPE), 188
subcutaneous delivery method, 111
subdermal delivery method, 111
subunit vaccines, 72–75
Sudden Infant Death Syndrome (SIDS), 119
superinfections, 38–40
supplements, immune system and, 224
swelling, as side effect, 113–114
swine flu
  hesitancy toward vaccines and, 190
  overview, 21
symptoms
  colds, 35–40
    causes, 34–35
    defined, 34
    flu vs., 36
    strep throat vs., 37–38
    whooping cough vs., 36–37

symptoms *(continued)*
  COVID-19, 44–46
  dehydration, 101
  Ebola, 28
  hepatitis, 89, 91
  HIV, 24
  live pathogen vaccines, 71
  measles, 25
  meningitis, 98
  mononucleosis, 202
  noroviruses, 24–25
  rotavirus, 130
  systemic, 106
  thrombocytopenia, 120
  varicella, 27
  West Nile virus, 208
  Zika virus, 209

T

teenagers, vaccines for, 143–144
testing
  for COVID-19, 47
  ingredients, 13
  vaccines, 75–77
tetanus
  overview, 63, 131
  vaccines for
    adults, 150–151, 155
    children, 131–132, 142–143
    effectiveness, 87
    rashes, 113
thimerosal
  hesitancy toward vaccines and, 189
  mercury and, 109
  overview, 108
Third Plague Pandemic, 215
thrombocytopenia, as side effect, 120
timing of vaccination
  cancer and, 162
  flu, 154
  hepatitis, 129
toxins
  from bacteria, 59
  overview, 11–14

toxoid vaccines, 14, 73–74
2-phenoxyethanol, 109
type A influenza virus, 19–21
type B influenza virus, 21
type C influenza virus, 21
type D influenza virus, 22
typhoid
  overview, 64
  travel and, 159
  vaccines for, 81
Tyrell, David, 32

V

Vaccine Adverse Event Reporting System (VAERS)
  overview, 116, 180
  website for, 181
vaccine derived polio virus (cVDPV), 183
vaccines
  acellular
    defined, 58
    pertussis, 88
  for adults
    catching up on missed childhood vaccines, 160
    COVID-19, 149–150
    diphtheria, 150–151, 155
    herpes zoster, 151–153
    influenza, 148–149, 153–155
    pertussis, 150–151, 155
    pneumococcus, 99–100, 156
    during pregnancy, 156–157
    shingles, 151–153
    Tdap, 150–151, 155
    tetanus, 150–151, 155
    whooping cough, 150–151, 155
  after organ transplants, 164–165
  for anthrax, 82
  antibiotics vs., 64–66
  avoiding, 161–165
  benefits of, 8–9
  for children
    diphtheria, 131–132, 142–143
    hepatitis A, 140
    hepatitis B, 128–129
    Hib, 132

HPV, 141–142
importance of, 127
influenza, 133–134
IPV, 132–133
laws, 140–141
measles, 137
MenACWY, 142
mumps, 137
myths regarding, 181–184
PCV13, 134
pertussis, 131–132, 142–143
pneumococcus, 100–101
rotavirus, 129–130
rubella, 138
scheduling, 144–146
Tdap, 131–132, 142–143
tetanus, 131–132, 142–143
varicella, 139–140
whooping cough, 131–132, 142–143
clinical phases of, 76–77
conjugate
MenACWY, 98
overview, 73
costs of, 75–76
for COVID-19
adults, 149–150
ingredients in, 171–172
overview, 50–53
reactions to, 170–173
delivery methods, 110–111
for diphtheria
adults, 150–151, 155
children, 131–132, 142–143
effectiveness, 86–87
rashes, 113
efficacy of, 78–80
for encephalitis, 197
for flu
adults, 148–149, 153–155
children, 133–134
effectiveness, 93–95
history of, 82
yearly, 15
for hepatitis, 89–91
for herpes zoster

adults, 151–153
overview, 102–104
hesitancy toward, 176–179
for Hib
children, 132
overview, 88–89
history of, 80–83
for HPV
children, 141–142
teenagers, 143
inactivated
overview, 72
polio, 132–133
for influenza
adults, 148–149, 153–155
children, 133–134
effectiveness, 93–95
history of, 82
yearly, 15
ingredients, 10–11
2-phenoxyethanol, 109
adjuvants, 10–11, 106–108, 166–167
aluminum, 108
antibiotics, 110
antigens, 10, 19–20, 47, 58, 93, 106–107, 127, 184
in COVID-19 vaccine, 171–172
eggs, 11, 110, 167
formaldehyde, 110, 189
gelatin, 109, 166
latex, 117, 167–168
in Moderna vaccine, 172
myths regarding, 188–189
in Pfizer vaccine, 171–172
phenol, 109
preservatives, 11, 106, 108, 166–167
production materials, 11, 106, 110
stabilizers, 11, 106, 109, 166–167
testing, 13
thimerosal, 108–109
yeast, 167
limiting, 161–165
live pathogen, 70–72, 164
for measles
children, 137
effectiveness, 95–97

vaccines *(continued)*
    hesitancy toward, 177
    history of, 82–83
    rashes, 113
  for meningococcus
    MenACWY, 142–143
    overview, 97–98
  mRNA
    COVID-19, 50–52, 171
    overview, 14, 74
  for mumps
    children, 137
    effectiveness, 95–97
    history of, 82–83
    rashes, 113
  myths regarding
    autism, 187–188
    cause of disease, 185–186
    causing death, 180–181
    causing disease, 185–186
    children, 181–184
    ingredients, 188–189
    natural immunity, 186–187
    overloading immune
      system, 184
    side effects, 180–181
  nucleic acid, 74
    COVID-19, 50–52, 171
    overview, 74
  overview, 9–11, 85
  for pertussis
    adults, 150–151, 155
    children, 131–132,
      142–143
    effectiveness, 88
  for pneumococcus
    adults, 99–100, 156
    effectiveness, 98–101
  for polio, 132–133
    history of, 82, 182
    inventors, 195–196
  polysaccharide, 59, 73
  protein-based, 73
  reactogenic
    defined, 52
    overview, 114
    shingles, 103

    recalling, 189–190
  for rubella
    children, 138
    effectiveness, 95–97
    history of, 82–83
    rashes, 113
  scheduling
    importance of, 15–16
    overview, 144–146
  for shingles
    adults, 151–153
    overview, 102–104
  SIDS and, 119
  for smallpox
    Inventor, 193–194
    overview, 80–81
  subunit, 72–75
  taking precautions before, 169–170
  for teenagers, 143–144
  testing
    clinical trial phases, 75–77
    overview, 13
  for tetanus
    adults, 150–151, 155
    children, 131–132, 142–143
    effectiveness, 87
    rashes, 113
  timing
    cancer and, 162
    hepatitis, 129
    influenza, 154
  toxoid
    defined, 14
    overview, 73–74
  types of
    cancer and, 162–163
    overview, 70–75
  for typhoid, 81
  for varicella
    children, 139–140
    effectiveness, 85–86, 95–97
    history of, 83
    rashes, 113
  viral vector
    COVID-19, 51
    defined, 14
    overview, 74–75

whole-pathogen, 70–72

for whooping cough

adults, 150–151, 155

children, 131–132, 142–143

effectiveness, 88

for yellow fever, 81

vaccinia, 185

VAERS (Vaccine Adverse Event Reporting System)

overview, 116, 180

website for, 181

variants

COVID-19, 48–49

flu, 82

varicella

hospitalization for, 86

overview, 26–27

R0, 85

vaccines for

children, 139–140

effectiveness, 85–86, 95–97

history of, 83

rashes, 113

variola, 29

variolation

defined, 178

smallpox and, 80

VHF (viral hemorrhagic fever), 28

Vibrio cholerae

overview, 60

pandemic caused by, 214

viral hemorrhagic fever (VHF), 28

viral vector vaccines

COVID-19 vaccine, 14

Johnson & Johnson vaccine, 51

overview, 74–75

virions, 17

viruses.

adenoviruses

cancer and, 39

COVID-19, 51

symptoms, 35

attenuated, 71

bacteria vs., 11–14, 57–58

baculovirus, 93

baculoviruses, 93

CMV, 200–201

coronaviruses

causes of, 34–35

defined, 34

identifying, 32–33

MERS, 41–42

RSV

SARS, 40–41

symptoms, 35–40

COVID-19

cancer and, 163

coping with, 56

detecting infection, 46–49

herd immunity, 53–55

long, 46

overview, 14–15

pandemic, 42–44, 218

protecting against, 55–56

risks for hospitalization, 45–46

symptoms, 44–45

testing for, 47

vaccination after infection, 173

vaccine ingredients, 171–172

vaccine reactions, 170–173

vaccines for, 50–53, 149–150

variants of, 48–49

coxsackieviruses, 35

cVDPV, 183

cytomegalovirus, 200–201

defined, 17

Ebola, 27–29

EBV, 201–202

enteroviruses

overview, 22–23

symptoms, 35

hepatitis

A, 140

B, 128–129

C, 202–203

vaccines for, 89–91

HIV

antiretroviral treatment, 204–205

finding cure for, 204–205

overview, 24–25

pandemic, 217–218

viruses *(continued)*

  HPV, 143

    overview, 92

    vaccines for, 141–143

  HSV, 203–204

  human metapnuemoviruses, 35

  influenza

    bird flus, 20, 200

    cancer and, 163

    colds vs., 36

    coping with, 56

    overview, 18–22

    pandemics, 215–217

    swine flu, 21, 190

    vaccines for, 15, 82, 93–95, 133–134, 148–149, 153–155

    variants, 82

  measles

    overview, 25–26

    vaccines for, 82–83, 95–97, 113, 137

  metapnuemoviruses, 35

  noroviruses, 23–24

  overview, 11–14, 18

  parainfluenza, 35

  rhinoviruses

    overview, 22–23

    symptoms, 35

  rotavirus

    in children, 129–130

    overview, 101–102

  RSV

    overview, 207

    symptoms, 35–36

  smallpox, 29

  toxins vs., 11–14

  vaccinia, 185

  varicella

    overview, 26–27

    vaccines for, 83, 85–86, 113, 139–140

  variola, 29

  West Nile virus, 208

  Zika virus, 209

vitamins, 224

W

West Nile virus, 208

wet stage of Ebola, 28

wheal, 111

WHO (World Health Organization)

  ingredients approved by, 13

  pandemics and

    COVID-19, 42, 218

    swine flu, 21

    Third Plague Pandemic, 215

  smallpox and, 29

  vaccines schedules and, 146

whole-pathogen vaccines, 70–72

whooping cough

  colds vs., 36–37

  overview, 62

  vaccines for

    adults, 150–151, 155

    children, 131–132, 142–143

    effectiveness, 88

World Health Organization (WHO)

  ingredients approved by, 13

  pandemics and

    COVID-19, 42, 218

    swine flu, 21

    Third Plague Pandemic, 215

  smallpox and, 29

  vaccines schedules and, 146

Wright, Almroth, 81

Y

yeast, 167

yellow fever

  travel and, 158

  vaccines for, 81

Yersinia pestis, 213

Z

Zika virus, 209

zinc, 224

Zostavax, 103

About the Authors

Megan Coffee, MD, PhD (DPhil), is an infectious disease doctor in New York City. She has worked on epidemics around the world from Ebola to cholera to COVID and has also run a TB program in Haiti with the nonprofit Ti Kay. She is on faculty at New York University Grossman School of Medicine and is an infectious disease physician at Bellevue Hospital in New York. She went to Harvard University for college and medical school and received her doctoral degree from Oxford University, before training in Internal Medicine at Massachusetts General Hospital and in Infectious Diseases at the University of California at San Francisco. She also teaches at Columbia University on outbreaks in low resource settings. She additionally works on computer models of infectious diseases to better predict and respond to epidemics.

Sharon Perkins has had the best of worlds, career-wise, spending 35-plus years as an RN, mostly working in maternal-child health, and writing professionally for over 20 years, including numerous *For Dummies* books. Her five children, two daughters-in-law, and one son-in-law make her proud every day, and her three beyond wonderful grandchildren are all growing up too quickly!

Dedication

Megan: To Dr. Larissa Lee.

Sharon: This book is dedicated to all the people who never had a chance to be vaccinated. And to my mom, who made darn sure we kids always got our shots, whether we wanted them or not!

Authors' Acknowledgments

Megan: I want to acknowledge all the nurses, doctors, and healthcare colleagues I have worked alongside around the world. Special thoughts for those who work where vaccines are not always easily accessible and for the patients they care for.

Thank you to all of those who worked on this project: Senior Acquisitions Editor Tracy Boggier, Development Editor Georgette Beatty, Managing Editor Kristie Pyles, and Sharon Perkins, my coauthor and wordsmith.

Sharon: Writing can be a lonely profession, but I've never found it so. Because I'd spend way too much time typing, left to my own devices, I appreciate the people in my life who give me a reason to get up and do something else. After living for years across the country, my mom, sister, and I spent the last five years living in close proximity. They were a huge part of my "fun" life for these past few years, and I thank them for it.

Of course, my children and grandchildren remain one of my main sources of fun and entertainment as well. There's nothing like spending time with family! Unless it's spending time with good friends. The friends I've made and remain connected with over 35 years in the workplace and outside can never be thanked enough for giving my life balance.

I thank every person I've helped take care of over these last three decades. As a nurse, especially in pediatric home health, your clients become a huge part of your life. It's been a true privilege to know so many great kids, as well as their parents and grandparents.

And one last group to thank — the editors and behind-the-scenes group at Wiley, including (this go-around) Senior Acquisitions Editor Tracy Boggier, Development Editor Georgette Beatty, and Managing Editor Kristie Pyles. And my coauthor Megan Coffee — I know it wasn't easy for you to write this during a pandemic! Thanks for hanging in there.

Publisher's Acknowledgments

Senior Acquisitions Editor: Tracy Boggier

Senior Managing Editor: Kristie Pyles

Project Manager and Development Editor: Georgette Beatty

Copy Editor: Christine Pingleton

Production Editor: Tamilmani Varadharaj

Cover Image: © ayo888/Getty Images